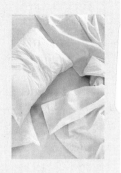

SINK INTO SLEEP

A Step-by-Step Workbook for Reversing Insomnia

Judith R. Davidson, PhD, CPsych

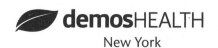

demosHEALTH

New York

Visit our website at www.demoshealth.com

ISBN: 978-1-936303-38-0
e-book ISBN: 978-1-617051-28-9
Acquisitions Editor: Noreen Henson
Compositor: diacriTech

Medical information provided by Demos Health, in the absence of a visit with a health care professional, must be considered as an educational service only. This book is not designed to replace a physician's independent judgment about the appropriateness or risks of a procedure or therapy for a given patient. Our purpose is to provide you with information that will help you make your own health care decisions.

The information and opinions provided here are believed to be accurate and sound, based on the best judgment available to the authors, editors, and publisher, but readers who fail to consult appropriate health authorities assume the risk of injuries. The publisher is not responsible for errors or omissions. The editors and publisher welcome any reader to report to the publisher any discrepancies or inaccuracies noticed.

Library of Congress Cataloging-in-Publication Data
CIP data is available from the Library of Congress.

Special discounts on bulk quantities of Demos Health books are available to corporations, professional associations, pharmaceutical companies, health care organizations, and other qualifying groups. For details, please contact:

Special Sales Department
Demos Medical Publishing, LLC
11 West 42nd Street, 15th Floor
New York, NY 10036
Phone: 800-532-8663 or 212-683-0072
Fax: 212-941-7842
E-mail: rsantana@demosmedpub.com

Printed in the United States of America by Hamilton Printing.
12 13 14 15 / 5 4 3 2 1

For Rick

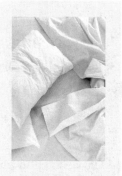

Table of Contents

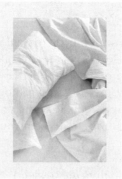

Foreword

I have worked with Dr. Judith Davidson as a colleague, fellow educator, and researcher in sleep for 12 years, on a wide range of sleep issues, including the subject of this book, insomnia. Her training in clinical psychology complements mine in physiology, and makes it particularly enjoyable to collaborate with her on activities such as team-teaching an undergraduate and a postgraduate course in sleep. Judith never rests on the topic of sleep, and continues to deepen her knowledge in the field by collaborating with international experts such as Dr. Charles Morin, knowledge that she shares with her peers, patients, and students. It's been a pleasure to work with, and learn from, Judith over the years.

Judith's extensive clinical and research experience has enabled her to provide insomnia sufferers with a practical guide to sleeping well. Insomnia is a significant burden to individuals, their family and society, affecting approximately 40% of adults 3 or more times a week. Her new book, *Sink Into Sleep*, encapsulates that knowledge in her own gracious style, and can teach insomnia sufferers powerful techniques for overcoming their own late night struggles.

Judith begins by clearly and succinctly describing the biology underlying sleep processes, giving the reader the basic understanding that is necessary to master the techniques of successful sleep. Age, being female, and genetics are known risk factors for insomnia, and each of these topics is discussed in this book. She also addresses key influences, such as the impact of various conditions including chronic pain, depression, cancer, and heart disease, as well as breathing disorders and movement disorders. Although the book focuses on nonpharmacological treatment for insomnia, she also outlines the pros and cons of sleep medications.

From laying the foundation by describing biological sleep processes, Judith guides the reader through 6 steps to solid sleep. The techniques she describes are grounded in research and evidence-based outcomes. The tools that she provides enable readers to self-monitor and measure their weekly progress toward optimizing their sleep. In one of her anecdotes, a man describes regaining sleep as being tapped by a "velvet hammer": Judith's calm, considered approach allows sufferers to beat the desperate frustration of seemingly perpetually elusive sleep.

For once, I am grateful when a book puts me to sleep, and I hope this book *Sink Into Sleep* does the same for you.

Helen S. Driver, PhD, RPSGT, DABSM
Past-President, Canadian Sleep Society
www.canadiansleepsociety.com
Sleep Disorders Laboratory
Kingston General Hospital and
Department of Medicine
Queen's University
Kingston, Ontario, Canada

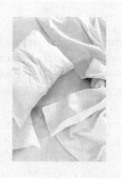

Preface

My career began in a sleep lab. I was hired in 1981 by Dr. Harvey Moldofsky to work in the sleep clinic at Toronto Western Hospital. A year earlier, I had taken a fascinating course, called The Psychology of Sleep, taught by Professors Alistair MacLean and John Knowles at Queen's University. This course inspired me to apply to every sleep laboratory I could locate. At that time, sleep labs were few and far between, and so I was fortunate to land a job in one.

I was involved in all of the day and night activities of the sleep lab, which included hooking people up with electrodes and putting them to bed so that we could see if they had a sleep disorder such as sleep apnea, periodic limb movements, narcolepsy, or unusual behaviors during sleep. We also did research studies with volunteers who agreed to have their brain waves and blood studied so we could look at the effects of sleep and sleep deprivation on the immune system. I realize now just how much I learned back then, in that lab. That experience turned out to be my stepping stone to many more years in the ever-expanding world of the science of sleep.

I have never strayed far from sleep. My master's thesis focused on the effects of sleep deprivation and naps on people's performance and mood. My PhD thesis was done with cancer patients. I surveyed 1,000 people with cancer to find out what types of sleep problems they experienced. About one-third of them reported sleep difficulty that occurred most nights and that affected their daytime functioning. By matching up the types of insomnia and the reported reasons for the sleep difficulty to the best available techniques, I developed a Sleep Therapy program for cancer patients. The program worked well to restore people's sleep; it also helped to reduce their fatigue. This was very encouraging. I then had the privilege of being a postdoctoral fellow with Dr. Charles Morin, a world leader in the field of insomnia, in Quebec City. Following that fellowship, I had a private psychology practice for a few years. People of all descriptions and health circumstances were coming for help with their insomnia. More recently, I have been providing Sleep Therapy in a family practice setting to patients who often have medical or emotional conditions.

Over the years it has become very clear to me that certain techniques reverse insomnia, regardless of whether we have cancer, chronic pain, heart disease, depression, anxiety, or any other human ailment. Dealing with insomnia when you have other health issues is just a variation on dealing with insomnia when that is your only problem.

These days, I focus on connecting people who have insomnia to effective treatments so they can sleep well, and so they know how to maintain their good sleep. A big part of this is trying to boost access to effective treatments, through the training of professionals, and spreading the word to the community at large, so that more people know about the techniques. It is why I have written this book. It is my sincere hope that this book provides you with what you need to sleep well. Be encouraged, even if you have had insomnia for many years, that the techniques that I will show you have been scientifically studied for years and they are effective for improving sleep. In fact, together, they are the best treatment for persistent insomnia.

One of the main concepts of this book was inspired by an encounter I had years ago with a tiny, elderly man at a cancer center. When I asked about his sleep, he told me that during his treatments for cancer, he had weeks and weeks of sleepless nights. However, just after the series of treatments ended, a wee angel had swept down and knocked him tenderly on the head with a velvet hammer, thus restoring his sleep from that point onward. I will not forget the twinkle in his eye and the smile that stretched from ear to ear. Sleep had found him. Indeed, sleep is something that we cannot actively search for, because in doing so, it evades us. Trying too hard to control sleep pushes it away. Rather, we have to make the circumstances conducive to sleep, and then relax, involve our minds in other things, and be delighted when it comes. This is the "velvet hammer" concept. The techniques in this book are designed to let your internal sleep–wake rhythms operate naturally, without interference. By relying on them, rather than over-thinking or trying to control sleep, you too will find that something changes, allowing the velvet hammer of sleep to descend.

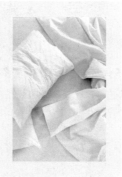

Acknowledgments

I am fortunate to have had encouragement and assistance from many people. A big smile and my heartfelt thanks go to Brenda Bass and Glenyss Turner, who both devoted hours to reading the book and offering helpful suggestions. Glenyss also entered and checked all the references. I am grateful to both of you for sharing your wisdom and talents. I wish to acknowledge the support of Queen's University and Queen's University Faculty Association who provided a grant from the Scholarly and Professional Development Fund when I began this project. Thank you to the following people for reviewing sections of the book: Aïda Sulcs, Jim Willis, Bruce Beninger, Helen Driver, Peet de Villiers, Richard J. Beninger, Alice Layton Falchetto, Jane Lapointe, Hugh Ryan, Barbara Muirhead, Theresa Krug, Cathy Hollington, Marcia Bryant, Bonnie Ramsay, Clint Flood, and Sylvia Bass-West. You each know what you contributed and I appreciate every little bit. Eric Brousseau's skillful work on the design of the forms allowed me to pilot test them to make sure they worked for readers. Finally, I've benefited from the continued stability and occasional frivolity provided by my running buddies. Thank you everyone.

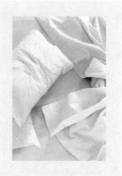

SINK INTO SLEEP

A Step-by-Step Workbook for Reversing Insomnia

Hope

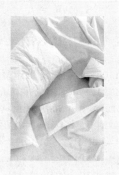

Chapter 1

Will This Book Help You?

You may be at your wits' end, thinking that you have tried everything to sleep better, and nothing has really worked. Or you may be optimistic, believing that there are things you have not yet tried that may improve your sleep. Or you may be somewhere in between. Wherever you are, it's okay to be there. The strategies in the next chapters work even, or especially(!), if you are a bit skeptical to begin with.

If you are "at your wits' end"—hang in there. Just by opening this book, you are demonstrating hope and a belief that things can change for the better. All that's needed is having your mind open to the possibility that your sleep will improve. However, you don't need to be gung-ho about it. In fact, it is better if you are somewhat relaxed and take on an observer's state of mind. If you are thinking, "That's not me! I can't relax," just have a bit of blind faith that your body and mind do have the capacity for good sleep, and that by using some specific techniques, you will encounter evidence of this.

If you are "optimistic"—then, good for you! Hang on to that style of thinking. You can use your energy and enthusiasm to design your own sleep program. You need to have a bit of patience, though, as this is not an overnight fix for your sleep. Rest assured that you will see positive results as you consistently apply the techniques.

If you are "somewhere in between"—not completely discouraged and not overly enthusiastic—you may be in the best position to benefit from sleep strategies. You have energy to try some things, but in a somewhat experimental way, with an ability to work with "what is" and an openness to discovering how sleep therapy works and to identifying the techniques that work best for you.

THE TECHNIQUES WORK

Years of research have revealed that certain techniques reliably lead to improved quality and quantity of sleep and increased satisfaction with sleep. Together these techniques can be called "cognitive behavioral therapy for insomnia" (which I will now call CBT-I). In the mid-1990s two important reports were published on these techniques. These reports were based on "meta-analyses." In a meta-analysis, the research data from many studies of a given treatment are combined to provide the overall story on the treatment's usefulness. In these particular meta-analyses, the authors reviewed studies that had compared CBT-I techniques with no treatment or with a placebo treatment. These two meta-analyses were carried out independently, one in North America and one in Australia. It was exciting when the results came out (they were published within months of each other). The reports reached similar conclusions: CBT-I techniques produced significant improvements in sleep for people with insomnia. More exciting was the evidence that sleep improvements were well maintained, and sometimes enhanced, 6–8 months after people had learned the techniques.

More recent reviews and clinical practice guidelines have confirmed that there is sound scientific evidence for the effectiveness of CBT-I techniques. The research shows that people with persistent insomnia who use these techniques reduce their time awake in bed, reduce the number of awakenings, and increase their nightly sleep duration. People tend to like these techniques and ratings of sleep quality and satisfaction with sleep are enhanced by using them. In sum, the evidence is consistently positive for the effectiveness of these treatments. It is high time these techniques were widely accessible to people who need relief from insomnia.

IMPROVEMENTS ARE FASTER THAN YOU MIGHT THINK

Many people who need these techniques do not know about them. Family physicians are the health professionals who most often hear about sleep problems. But family physicians are very busy people; they usually do not have the time to learn or to support patients with sleep treatments other than drugs. They sometimes prescribe sleeping pills, also called hypnotic medication. Hypnotic medication is good for the short term only (up to 4 weeks). This book will show you how to deal with and overcome your insomnia if you have insomnia that has lasted *longer than 4 weeks*. The approaches I will suggest do not work overnight. However, it does not take long to see improvements in your sleep with CBT-I approaches. Most people in the clinic start sleeping better within 2 weeks of trying the techniques. After finding the combination of techniques that work best for their situation, they simply fine-tune them. The vast majority of people who use these techniques in the clinic no longer have insomnia after 5 weeks.

GOOD SLEEP CAN BE MAINTAINED

There is evidence that by using CBT-I approaches, people not only maintain their good sleep over time—the current research has followed people up to 2 years—but they often see their sleep continuing to improve! My experience is that once people understand their sleep problem and identify the combination of simple strategies that works for them, they remember and use these strategies when faced with transient sleep difficulty months and years later. By doing so, they prevent relapses into full-blown insomnia.

Let me now address a few concerns that are quite common when people first consider CBT-I.

YOU ARE NOT A HOPELESS CASE—THERE ARE NO HOPELESS CASES

People sometimes feel that their particular case of insomnia is hopeless. This idea is expressed by people who have had poor sleep for many years despite having tried "everything." First, let me say that even if you have had long-term insomnia these techniques still work. The research results are somewhat unclear about whether or not you will take a bit longer to improve your sleep, but is very clear that you can still benefit. In some of my research with insomnia expert Dr. Charles Morin, people arriving at his clinic had been experiencing sleep difficulty for an average of 11 years! People whose insomnia had persisted for years or decades have used these techniques very successfully.

Many people who come to the clinic have already tried various strategies to obtain better sleep. Usually they have tried very reasonable approaches like avoiding caffeine, a warm bath in the evening, relaxation recordings, music, yoga, cardiovascular exercise to tire themselves out, stretching, avoiding stimulating activities or television shows in the evening, their own relaxation exercise (such as counting sheep, deep breathing, progressive relaxation), and so on. One person was convinced that slowly stretching the whole body just before sleep, like a cat, promotes sleep. However, I have noticed that cats tend to stretch *after* rather than before sleeping. To be like a cat we would need to make three turns before settling down and then spend a few moments licking our feet! (Cats are certainly great sleepers and we can learn a lot about letting go from them.)

Even though such strategies may be helpful, they do not reverse chronic insomnia. These so-called "sleep hygiene" strategies may be helpful for people when they are feeling stressed and have situational insomnia but research has shown that they do not work for persistent insomnia. Many of the strategies of CBT-I are not yet well known but that will soon change. The effective strategies are the ones that I will introduce you to in the chapters ahead.

YOU ARE NOT TOO OLD TO START

This is not just an approach for young people. There is abundant evidence from research that middle-aged and older adults with insomnia benefit from CBT-I and that the beneficial effects endure. As we age we are more and more likely to have difficulties sleeping through the night. CBT-I improves sleep quality and reduces time awake during the night. It is also safer than using sleeping medications. Sleeping pills can cause side effects that are particularly worrisome for older people, including an increased risk of falls.

THERE PROBABLY ISN'T A CHEMICAL IMBALANCE

The cases where a chemical imbalance in the brain or a brain lesion produces poor sleep are rare. Although insomnia can accompany most illnesses, there are not many conditions that directly and specifically cause insomnia through a chemical imbalance. The closest thing might be a disease called "fatal familial insomnia" that causes inability to sleep. This is a genetically inherited prion (infectious protein) disease. The incidence of this disease is so rare that it is not documented; it is definitely less than 1 in 100,000 and probably less than 1 in 1 million. If you have this disease, you would have already turned yourself over to physicians for help. So, if you are reading this book, chances are that your sleep difficulty is not caused by a chemical imbalance. It is more likely related to factors that I outline in the chapters ahead and will therefore respond to CBT-I.

YOU'VE BEEN TAKING SLEEP MEDICATION. THAT'S OKAY

Research shows that the same CBT-I techniques work regardless of whether you are taking sleeping medication or not. Usually people's use of sleep medication decreases gradually over time as they use CBT-I and discover that they can sleep without the medication. If you have been taking prescribed sleep medications every night for more than 2 months, you might decide to slowly withdraw from the medication in consultation with your family physician. If so, it is very important that you do so in a gradual and planned way with medical guidance. This means over weeks and months. Otherwise there will be uncomfortable withdrawal symptoms including worsened insomnia.

YOU HAVE OTHER HEALTH OR MOOD ISSUES. THAT'S OKAY

If you are a normal human being, you have other problems besides trouble sleeping. Research shows that CBT-I is useful even if you have some mild to moderate symptoms of anxiety or depression, or some long-lasting medical problem like chronic pain or cancer. In fact, there is some evidence that people with coexisting health or mood conditions show greater improvements in their sleep with these techniques than do people who have "just" insomnia! Chapters 20 and 21 will describe how to tailor your program to your situation.

All that being said, there are some specific circumstances in which this Sleep Therapy program may not be enough to help your sleep.

CIRCUMSTANCES WHEN THIS BOOK MAY NOT BE ENOUGH

If you are severely depressed and have not received any treatment yet, you need to visit your family physician and get advice on the best available treatment. By severely depressed, I mean feeling so low that you are having difficulty getting out of bed every day, not functioning as usual, not able to go to work, or feeling hopeless or suicidal. You should know that there are effective treatments for depression, some involve medications, and some involve psychotherapy (e.g., cognitive behavioral therapy or interpersonal therapy). Your family physician is the first person to talk with about the options in your community.

Another situation in which you may need special support and assistance is bereavement. If someone close to you has recently died, then you are likely to be grieving and this needs time and special attention; it is not the best time to do this program. Furthermore, if you have experienced or witnessed an extremely traumatic event that has left you feeling vulnerable and jumpy, distressed or detached, and you have intense recollections, flashbacks, or nightmares related to the trauma, then you need to receive support from someone who understands trauma. Preliminary research indicates that CBT-I may help your disturbed sleep, but I suggest that you receive help from a trauma specialist first.

If you need alcohol or other non prescribed or street drugs in order to get through the day or if your use of these substances is interfering with your day-to-day functioning, then the CBT-I techniques will probably not be appropriate for you. That is because most, if not all, recreational drugs affect sleep directly and compromise people's ability to follow this program. If you are a smoker, the CBT-I techniques will probably help your sleep. However, I recommend for your own health and well-being that you consider a smoking cessation program. There is support in your community; start with your family physician or your local health unit. I would *not* recommend that you try to stop smoking or any other psycho-active substance at the same time as taking this sleep therapy program. Changing one behavior at a time is much more manageable.

If you are troubled by obsessions (have difficulty letting go of certain thoughts, impulses or images—ones that go around and around in your head or that pop into your mind when you don't want them there) or by compulsions (feeling compelled to do certain things over and over before you feel comfortable, such as checking, counting, pairing things up in your mind, washing your hands many more times than needed), you should know that there is help for these obsessive-compulsive symptoms. It would be wise to receive help for them first, before following this CBT-I program. Your family physician would be the place to start if you have not already received help.

If there is a medical condition that directly causes the insomnia, for example, untreated hyperthyroidism or acute, unrelenting pain due to a bone fracture or injury, then the insomnia will likely continue until the condition is treated or controlled. Also, certain medications such as corticosteroid medication can cause sleeplessness. If your insomnia started around the time of a new medication and it persists only with the medication, then discuss this with the physician who prescribed that medication, your family physician, or your pharmacist. They may suggest alterations to the dose, timing, or other factors that will allow you to return to good sleep.

Sometimes other sleep disorders masquerade as insomnia. These other sleep disorders have treatments of their own. Periodic limb movement disorder is a problem in which the person's legs twitch or make small jerks repetitively during sleep. This can disrupt sleep even if the person is unaware of the movements, and can cause an unsatisfying, light sleep. Many people who have restless legs syndrome—a restless feeling in the legs that urges them to walk or move around—also have periodic limb movement disorder. Sleep apnea is another fairly common sleep disorder, which involves loud snoring and a cessation of breathing for repeated periods of at least 10 seconds. This sleep disorder, especially when severe, can disrupt sleep, cause daytime sleepiness, and affect how you function at work, school or home. Sleep apnea needs to be treated so you can feel better. Treatment starts with visiting your family physician. He or she may refer you to a clinical sleep laboratory. There are effective treatments for these sleep disorders so it makes good sense to receive help for them. You can always come back to this CBT-I program if you still have insomnia after you have received help for the other sleep disorders.

By the way, there is NO NEED to go to a sleep laboratory if insomnia is your only sleep problem; that is, if you and your physician do not suspect another type of sleep disorder. You will probably not sleep in the lab—a finding that will confirm what you already know!

There is another sleep–wake disorder called "delayed sleep phase syndrome." This occurs when people's internal 24-hour rhythm of sleep and wakefulness is delayed compared to what they wish it were. These are people who have always been "night owls" and had trouble getting up in the morning. Young adults are more likely than middle-and older-age adults to experience this. If they had their choice they would have a late bedtime (e.g., 2–6 a.m.) and a late wake time (e.g., 10 a.m. to 1 p.m.). With this schedule their sleep would be normal. However, when they try to fit in with usual school or work hours and go to bed earlier than is normal for them, they take a long time to fall asleep and have great difficulty getting out of bed in the morning, even with several alarms. If this sounds like you, you will be more likely to benefit from a technique designed to advance your sleep rhythms than from CBT-I. A professional at a sleep clinic with expertise in the treatment of circadian rhythm disorders will be able to help you. This usually involves carefully sched-uled exposure to bright light.

If you are under a lot of pressure right now due to continuing stress at work or at home, or if there is ongoing conflict, you may want to seek support from a good counselor with these specific issues. If these issues are not resolved or at least stable, they may overwhelm your body's ability to benefit from CBT-I just now. If you travel frequently to different time zones, then some of the most powerful strategies will not be easy to carry out, so it is best to start this program when you are based at home.

Insomnia is very common among shift workers. Most shift schedules place a demand on your sleep–wake system. Some of these involve too much variation in your sleep timing for the techniques in this book to solve your sleep problem. This is true if you are working rotating shifts that require you to have very different bedtimes and rise times (for example, having to change your bedtime by 4 hours or more) within a 2-week period, or if you work permanent nights, and you shift to being awake during the day on your days off. These types of shift schedules are hard on the body and the mind, so look after yourself well. It is best to get help from an organization or circadian rhythm specialist with shift-work expertise. From them, you can learn strategies for sleeping as well as possible, and for maintaining other aspects of good health such as nutrition, exercise, recreation, connec-tions with family and your community, when you have shifting work and sleep schedules. For other types of shift work where there are no overnight shifts (for example, you move between day and evening shifts) and you can have a stable bedtime and rise time, then the techniques in this book should be helpful for you.

Finally, if you have too hectic a schedule that does not allow you time to focus on the program for a few minutes each day, then you may want to delay starting this program to a time when you can maximize your success with the strategies.

If all the issues in this section are either not relevant to you, or you have dealt with them, then it is time to move ahead into your insomnia treatment program! Let's start with some information about insomnia.

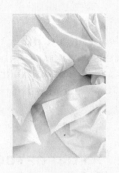

Chapter 2

What Is Insomnia?

It is normal to have a bout of poor sleep, light sleep, or seemingly no sleep at all under certain conditions. For example, if we have just lost someone due to illness, death, divorce, or a relationship break-up we will no doubt lose sleep. If there is conflict with people at work, too much work, difficult decisions to be made, arguments at home, or worries about children, we are bound to lose some sleep. If we have been exposed to trauma or dangerous situations where we feared for our lives then we are also likely to lose sleep or have a light, vigilant sleep. If we are thinking too much—studying, cramming for an exam, trying to solve complex problems—we may lose sleep. If we travel to another time zone, our sleep will take some days to adjust (this is "jet lag"). We usually have poor sleep on the first night in a strange bed (the so-called "first night effect"). If we are head over heels in love, then we are sometimes so excited that we hardly sleep. When we have babies who of course require care and feeding at night, we get very little sleep for several months. These are just some examples of situations when it is normal to not sleep well. The times when we are temporarily sleepless will depend to some extent on our individual predisposition to sleep disruption, our experience, and the aspects of life that stress us. For example, if job interviews stress you, as they do most of us, then it would not be surprising to have a poor night of sleep in anticipation of the interview.

When you look at these examples of sleepless nights from a biological perspective, it makes perfect sense that we can override our sleep drive when we need to be vigilant, to solve problems, to look after babies. It is an evolutionary adaptation that has allowed us to survive. Think of our ancient ancestors who had to be vigilant for predators or invaders. Similarly, the sleep behaviors of monkeys and apes, including the choice of sleeping sites and who gets up and out of the tree first in the morning, is very much determined by the need to protect the group against leopards and other predators. This ability to alter sleep behavior is crucial for survival. Likewise, in humans, the ability to stay awake is sometimes crucial and often useful. We want to maintain our ability to stay awake, or to awaken from sleep when there is a good reason. But when this happens repeatedly and needlessly, then this becomes a problem called insomnia.

THE DIFFERENCE BETWEEN A BOUT OF POOR SLEEP AND INSOMNIA

Insomnia is a complaint of difficulty falling asleep or staying asleep, or non restful sleep, that impairs our functioning or causes distress. It is frequently accompanied by fatigue. So, compared to a bout of poor sleep, insomnia is a sleep problem that takes on a life of its own. Basically it is persistent, unsatisfactory sleep that has daytime consequences. Although strictly speaking insomnia can be present for a very short time, it is usually only identified as such when it lasts for 1 month or longer.

I probably don't need to tell you that when sleep difficulty persists, we don't feel on top of the world. People with insomnia report low mood, irritability, poor concentration and memory, reduced physical well-being, and some difficulties interacting with other people. They also report having more fatigue-related car crashes than people without insomnia. People with insomnia seem to be able to perform mundane tasks of daily living but they tend to have less enjoyment of their activities and show less "cognitive flexibility"—they tend to think more narrowly and less creatively—than people who sleep well. Although they are often able to perform work and other activities well, everything feels like it takes more effort. In sum, when people don't sleep well for a long time, their mood, functioning, and quality of life are impaired.

Researchers who have observed people with insomnia over time—months or years—find that they are more likely than people without insomnia to use medical and mental health services. The exact reasons for this are not yet well understood. We know from several studies that insomnia increases the likelihood of subsequent development of clinical depression. The links between health, including mental health, and sleep are the subject of increasing numbers of research studies.

Often insomnia starts as a bout of poor sleep, triggered by an event or circumstance like the ones described at the beginning of this chapter. The bout turns into insomnia as other factors come into play. These factors are often behaviors or thoughts that hinder the arrival of sleep. It is *these* behaviors and thoughts that can be altered to help you get back to sleep. So the good news is that, regardless of the initial triggers of the sleep difficulty, insomnia can be reversed!

YOU ARE NOT ALONE

Although being awake in the middle of the night can be isolating, you should know that each night there are many other people on the planet who are wide awake. At least 1 in

10 people in your time zone will be awake at the same time due to insomnia. As many as 25% of the North American population report sleeping problems and about 10% have chronic sleep issues. This is a substantial portion of the population.

It might also help to think about all the night workers out there. For example, consider all the people in your time zone who are keeping the hospitals, care facilities, and factories running at night. In addition, you can think about all the people on Earth who are in more easterly time zones who are already "up and at it." You may be the only one awake in your house in the middle of the night, but you are definitely not the only one awake!

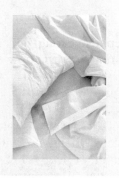

Chapter 3

Some Reassuring News

As insomnia develops, you may start to worry about not sleeping. One of my tennis friends had a stressful management position over which she started to lose sleep. She then feared that the lack of sleep would negatively affect her work performance. This made it even more difficult for her to sleep because the thought of underperforming increased her anxiety. You can see how this can become a cycle of worry and sleeplessness.

Let me go over some of the common worries that are linked to insomnia. By examining these topics in the light of day, rather than ruminating during a sleepless night, we achieve a more balanced view of our sleep problem and its effects. Stressful thoughts at night have a way of expanding to fill the dark spaces around us. The following information will help to bring your sleep-related worries down to earth.

OH NO, I'M NOT GETTING 8 HOURS OF SLEEP! HOW MUCH SLEEP SHOULD I BE GETTING?

People often ask me "How much sleep should I be getting?" or "How much sleep do we need?" They are usually looking for the answer to be a certain number of hours per night. Expecting the answer to be in hours is somewhat like asking "How much food do we need?" and expecting the answer to be in kilograms! If someone asked you how much food we humans need, would you say "3 pounds per day?" Not likely. Rather, you might say "It depends." It depends on the person's metabolism, how much energy he or she has expended that day, how old the person is, what time of day it is, what type of food it is, how nutritious it is, how hungry the person is, and so on. Why then, do we so often hear "We need 8 hours of sleep a night"? The need for sleep, like eating, depends on many factors. It depends on individual differences in sleep duration, our age, how active we were that day, how much sleep we got the night before, how sleepy we are, what type of sleep we achieve, its quality, and what time of day or night we go to bed.

The range of sleep durations among individuals is wide, just as there is a wide range of heights and shoe sizes; some people get along fine with 4 hours and some with 10 hours. In North America, the average duration of sleep is between 7 and 8 hours per night. However, this is just the *average*. A substantial proportion of people (about 25%–30% of the population) sleep 6 hours or less and a sizable proportion (10%–15%) sleep 9 hours or more. Also, it is important to know that our sleep duration changes throughout our life-span. As we age, we get less and less sleep. For example, someone who got 8 hours per night as a 20 year old may now be getting 6 hours at age 60. I'll discuss some of the reasons for this decline in sleep duration with age later (Chapters 18 and 19). Other things that affect sleep duration will be discussed along the way but I think you see the point, that the optimal duration of sleep is highly individual and depends on many factors. In a nutshell, the amount of sleep that *you* need is the amount that allows *you to feel rested and alert during the day*, whatever that duration is at this point in your life. You will discover how to estimate your optimal sleep duration as you proceed with the program in this book, and it will not necessarily be 8 hours!

ARE WE A "SLEEP-DEPRIVED SOCIETY?"

A *New York Times* headline in 1994 read "Health Alarm for a Sleep-Deprived Society." This is an example of media stories that stick in our minds about our society having a chronic sleep debt. The story goes that since the advent of the light bulb we have been getting less and less sleep! This is because our 24-hour activities, televisions, electronic devices, and modern busy lifestyles push sleep to dangerously short durations. Is this really true? Let's look at the question whether sleep duration is decreasing from decade to decade. Some research studies *have* found a trend for reduced sleep. For example, a study from Finland that examined the sleep duration reported by people from 1972 to 2005, found a reduction of 5.5 minutes every decade. The National Sleep Foundation in the United States, which does a telephone survey of 1,000 Americans every year, found a trend for the average sleep duration to decrease over time, amounting to a reduction of 18 minutes over the past decade. However, several other surveys have found that the average sleep duration has *not* gone down significantly. For example, a study from Great Britain found very little difference between sleep durations reported in the late 1960s and those in 2003. A recent, carefully done study from the United States did not find obvious evidence of shortened sleep over the years 1975 to 2006.

So, the story about reduced sleep durations over the decades is questionable. What we *do* see clearly in sleep duration studies is that long work hours are associated with short sleep, regardless of the decade. For example, full time workers are more likely than part-time workers to have short sleep. People who have high job demands and long hours (e.g., over 55 hours per week) are more likely to have short sleep that people who work regular hours (35–40 hours per week).

What about further back, say a century or two ago? It is difficult to know how long people slept in comparison to today because we must rely on anecdotal and non-standardized records. Before the widespread availability of electricity in the Western world, our sleep, work, and meal times would have depended more on patterns of natural light and darkness. Sleep duration probably varied widely by occupation, wealth (which determined whether you could afford candles, oil lamps, and other artificial light sources), latitude, and season. Although we cannot be sure about the average duration of sleep over the centuries, we can speculate that sleep duration was more related than it is now to seasonal changes in the timing of dusk and dawn, and the weather. There is some historical evidence that people in pre-industrial Europe had a "first sleep" (starting some time between sun down and midnight), were awake for a time in the middle of the night, and then had a "second sleep" early in the morning. Despite having two sleeps, it seems people did *not* achieve more or better sleep than what we get now. These days, our sleep duration is less related to our natural environment, and more related to the amount of work we do. I don't think we need to sound any alarms.

SO WHAT? DOES IT REALLY MATTER IF WE DON'T GET ENOUGH SLEEP?

We Become Tired and Irritable But We Can Function

When we don't get enough sleep we are likely to be grouchy. We are also likely to feel tired. Things feel a lot harder to do. A study by Dr. Gary Zammitt in New York City found that people with insomnia described low mood—feeling unhappy and having less interest in being with other people. They reported poor concentration, tiredness, mental slowness, and lethargy. They also felt accident-prone and clumsy. The good news is that, although things seem a lot harder, research shows that people with insomnia can function quite well. Their performance has been measured numerous times on a variety of tasks, such as reaction time, concentration, short-term memory, and motor tasks (those requiring movement). The vast majority of tasks are done just as well by people with insomnia as by good sleepers. However, people with insomnia feel that things are harder to do and require more exertion. They often feel that they haven't done as well as they would have liked, or as well as they actually have. All this suggests that we can usually get the job done—whether it be school work, house work, or job work—although we may feel that it takes extra effort. We are functional, but tired, sad, and irritable. No doubt about the irritability; it is a frequent companion of insomnia!

We May Feel Run-Down But Insomnia Does Not Make Us Sick

Some people worry that they will get sick because of poor sleep. Studies of sleep and the immune system—our body's capacity to snuff out invading organisms and fight off disease—are complex because there are many types of immune functions and many ways to measure them. You might think that we are more likely to catch a cold after losing sleep but this has *not* been found in sleep deprivation research. Contrary to popular belief, it appears that sleep deprivation is accompanied by *enhanced* immunity in the short term. This is believed to be a beneficial phenomenon that protects us from immediate dangers. For example, in our ancestral days, it may have allowed us to stay awake overnight to escape from predators, and to stay healthy during this period.

On the other hand, relentless long-term sleep deprivation probably does affect immunity: Animal studies show us that the immune system can fail after severe sleep deprivation over weeks. However, this type of severe sleep deprivation is not experienced by animals or humans in real life. So, there is no need to concern yourself with this extremely rare situation (see fatal familial insomnia, which I mentioned in Chapter 1).

Sleep loss of any duration can be accompanied by a heightened physiological stress response, including the release of stress hormones adrenalin and cortisol, but any link between this stress response and disease is not well understood. There have only been a very few studies of immune factors in people with insomnia. These have found some shifts in levels and activity of some immune system cells, but there is no clear evidence to date that insomnia or sleep loss makes us more susceptible to infection or disease. Certainly, one night of sleep loss does not significantly or obviously impair our health.

You may be saying—well what about all the nights of poor sleep I have had over the past 30 years?!! Surely the accumulation of sleepless nights has an effect on my functioning and health. Well, there is some evidence that *shortened sleep* over several days leads to some impairments in reaction time and short-term memory tasks. It may also alter the body's ability to metabolize glucose, which can make people more prone to weight gain and diabetes. However, this research is based on normal sleepers, healthy young people, who have their sleep cut short for several nights in a row. Insomnia is not the same thing as shortened sleep. With insomnia, as I said earlier: "We become tired and irritable but we can function." That pretty well sums it up. Very few research studies of insomnia have found obvious impairment in the ability to perform mental or physical activities. So, if chronic insomnia has negative effects on performance and health, those effects are not obvious.

We Have Some Control Over This Moment Only

You can also let go of worries about your past years of insomnia and concerns about future nights by realizing that *you can only have some control over the night that is here*. Worry about past or future nights serves no purpose other than impeding sleep tonight. You can tell yourself that this one night of sleep, even if it is poor, will not have devastating consequences on your daytime functioning or health. You can also reassure yourself that by using the techniques in this book you will be doing the best thing to improve your sleep now.

Our Sleep Rebounds

When we lose sleep one night, we can recover most of what we've lost the next time we sleep. Studies in which people are deprived of all sleep for one or more nights show that recovery sleep is a long, deep sleep. When people are selectively deprived of either deep "slow wave" sleep or rapid eye movement (REM) sleep (see Appendix A), they do not necessarily regain the duration of lost sleep on the following night. However, their sleep systems enter these stages earlier and with greater intensity on the following night. So, relax; if you lose some sleep on one night, your body has built-in mechanisms to restore it.

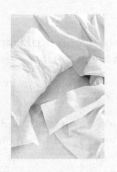

Chapter 4

Sleep Hygiene: What It Is and Why You Probably Don't Need It!

"**H**ygiene" means "principles of maintaining health; the practice of these" (Concise Oxford Dictionary, 1982). In Greek mythology, there was a goddess called Hygeia, the daughter of Ascelpius, the god of medicine. She was the goddess of health, and her name is the origin of our word "hygiene." In the strict sense "sleep hygiene rules" are tips for maintaining good sleep health. They include things that your grandmother may have told you, such as don't eat a big meal before you go to bed.

In my experience, people with persistent insomnia don't need these tips BECAUSE THEY ALREADY KNOW THEM. And they have already used them and found that these tips have not been enough to reverse their sleep problem. The research concurs: Sleep hygiene alone is not effective for chronic insomnia.

So, why am I including sleep hygiene in this book? I thought I should at least mention these tips because people do expect to see them in a book about sleep. Also, it may be a refreshing relief for you to see these tips tossed out the window. We are tossing them out the window, not because they are unhelpful, but because they are insufficient to reverse persistent insomnia. These are the types of recommendations or information "bites" that you see printed in magazine how-to articles. They may be helpful for people who usually sleep well or those who have situational insomnia in order to prevent further problems. By following them, one certainly eliminates some of the factors that can interfere with sleep. However, if you have been dealing with insomnia for a while, I'll bet you are already doing these things.

- Make your bedroom conducive to sleep. Consider the comfort of your bed, the air temperature, and levels of noise and light. *I'm sure you've thought of these things.*

- Minimize interference with your sleep by your bed partner, children, or pets. *This is important but more easily said than done!*

- Caffeine is a stimulant and should be discontinued 6 hours before bedtime. Know the foods, drink, and medications that contain caffeine. *I'm sure you already know that coffee, tea, cola, and dark chocolate all contain quite a bit of caffeine. You may have already cut out caffeine in the afternoon and evening.*

- Nicotine (e.g., from cigarettes) is a stimulant and should be avoided near bedtime. *There are many more health reasons to avoid smoking but this is the sleep-related one.*

- A light snack may be sleep-inducing but a heavy meal close to bedtime interferes with sleep. Avoid consuming chocolate, large amounts of sugar, and excessive fluids close to bedtime. *This is probably what Grandma told you.*

- Do not exercise vigorously within 3–4 hours of bedtime. *You are probably not doing gymnastics at 11 p.m. I suppose you might be playing hockey that late if that is the only ice time you can get.*

- Regular exercise in the late afternoon may deepen sleep. *You are probably aware of the positive effects of exercise on your mental and physical health. It is possible that you did not know about this relationship between the timing of exercise and sleep. A brisk walk or some cardiovascular exercise on a regular basis in the late afternoon may be helpful for your sleep but it may not be enough to reverse persistent insomnia.*

- Take time to relax and wind down in the evening prior to going to bed. *Don't work intensively on a project that's due tomorrow and then expect to drop off to sleep immediately. That makes sense.*

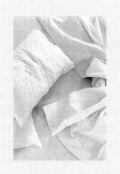

Chapter 5

Sleep Therapy: What It Is and Why You Need It

At the very beginning of this book I introduced you to something called cognitive behavioral therapy for insomnia, or CBT-I. This is the set of techniques that has been shown to be effective for relieving persistent insomnia and that form the foundation of this book. "Sleep Therapy" is the term I use for the specific program laid out here, which combines the most powerful and effective components of CBT-I. These techniques are relatively unknown now, but that's about to change. As a sleep researcher and clinician, I know these are the most reliable and effective techniques we have available to reverse persistent insomnia and that's exactly why you need them.

Let me tell you what to expect. Sleep Therapy starts with looking at what your sleep is like now. This is a crucial part of the program because this information will inform subsequent strategies. The first part of the program, called FIRST THINGS FIRST, involves recording your sleep using sleep diaries to assess the nature of your insomnia. You will then do some simple calculations to determine how much sleep you are getting now, and how "efficient" or solid your sleep is. You will also check to see if and how factors like alcohol, sleep medication, or naps may be affecting your nighttime sleep.

After you have looked at your current sleep patterns, you will move on to the second part of the program, called SOLVING YOUR INSOMNIA. Here, you will learn how to uncover, or rediscover, the biological processes that allow you to sleep. I will show you how to tailor your bedtime and rise time in order to get solid sleep, and how to associate your bed with great sleep. The procedures will be summarized in Six Steps to Solid Sleep, the main techniques of Sleep Therapy. You will monitor your progress, using sleep diaries, and learn how to make adjustments to your bedtime as you start to sleep well. After you have used the Sleep Therapy techniques for about 3 weeks, you will step back and evaluate if you still have insomnia or not. Most people experience vastly improved sleep by that point. In case you are one of the many people who has an active, racing mind that interferes with your ability to fall asleep, I will then show you how to move your mind into a state that is more conducive to having sleep arrive, to having the velvet hammer descend. So let's begin.

First Things First

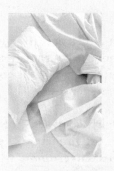

Chapter 6

Measuring Your Sleep Problem—Keeping a Sleep Diary

The most useful and efficient way of starting your sleep program is by understanding your current sleep-wake patterns. This way you can match your particular situation to a plan that will allow you to see your sleep improve as quickly as possible. As I was preparing this book, my friend Julie was having sleep difficulty. In fact, she had been struggling with insomnia for several years and it had gotten worse over the past year. She was waking up several times each night, often with menopausal hot flashes. After each arousal she would be awake for several minutes to hours. Occasionally, she was waking up much earlier in the morning than she wanted to. Also, over the past year she had started to have some trouble falling asleep at her bedtime on certain nights. She decided to try Sleep Therapy and to go though my draft book, chapter by chapter. She agreed for me to follow her progress and to use her calculations and experiences as examples for future readers. I will use Julie's situation as an example that you can refer to as we proceed from here. Thank you, Julie.

All right, let's start with the measurement of your sleep. The standard measurement tool for insomnia is the "sleep diary." Sleep diaries are not really diaries, but simple logs, based on your recollection of your last night's sleep. Because you are the expert on your insomnia, you are the best person to report on each night's sleep in order to measure your sleep problem. As I mentioned in Chapter 1, you do not need to go to a sleep laboratory unless your physician suspects another type of sleep disorder, such as a problem of excessive sleepiness or breathing disorders during sleep. In fact, people with insomnia who go to sleep labs usually have trouble sleeping in the lab, which simply confirms their insomnia.

Each morning's recordings take 2 minutes or less to do. Do it when you first wake up—as soon as your vision clears, your hand–eye coordination allows you to pick up a pen, and as soon as your mind is alert enough to know what is going on. Most people find that this is not a difficult task; some people even enjoy it.

Although you will probably have a fairly good sense of what time you went to bed and what time you got up in the morning, you will probably have only a fuzzy idea of what happened in between. That's okay. You only need to *estimate* what happened in between. For example, there is no way you can tell how long it took you to fall asleep exactly. You were drifting into a less-conscious state at the time and so, of course, it is hard to say precisely when that happened. Likewise, the number of times you woke up may not be clear, let alone the duration of those awakenings. Again, don't worry about this. You can "guess-timate." Avoid looking at the clock during the night; checking the clock increases alertness and hinders sleep. If you have a clock on your bedside table, turn it away from you. If you have a cell phone or other electronic device that you use for keeping track of the time, put it away, preferably in another room. Your rough estimate of the times and durations is all that is required. Research and experience tells us this is perfectly adequate for the job at hand.

In order to get familiar with your sleep–wake patterns, you will need to record at least 1 week's worth of sleep diaries, representing 7 nights, before you try any of the therapeutic techniques. This initial measurement of your sleep will provide you with a "baseline" measure. This is important information on which you will be basing your program of sleep improvement. Let's get started with your very first sleep diary.

LOGGING YOUR SLEEP WITH A SLEEP DIARY

At the end of this chapter you will see a blank sleep diary, labeled BASELINE. Feel free to photocopy this. The diary has enough room for you to track your sleep for 7 nights.[1] You will see that the top section of the sleep diary is for date information. Then there is a section called "Sleep timing." This consists of 7 questions about the timing of your sleep. The next tab is "Sleep quality" with a single question. Then you will see the bottom section with headings for naps, alcohol, and sleep medication.

Note that there are 7 vertical columns, one for each night of the week. Complete a column *each morning*, when your sleep is fresh in your memory.

- Start with *Sleep Diary for the Week of*: Record the month and day (and year if you want) of the first night of the week being reported on. For example, if you begin to fill in your sleep diary on September 21 about last night's sleep, you would enter September 20.

- For *Day of the Week* put in MON, TUES, WED, THURS, FRI, SAT, or SUN, depending on which night you are reporting on. For example, if you are starting on a Friday morning to report on Thursday night's sleep you would put "THURS" in the space at

---

[1] If your sleep varies a lot from week to week, or you don't think that 1 week will adequately represent your sleep, then you will want to keep sleep diaries for 2 weeks (14 nights). Photocopy the blank sleep diary at the end of this chapter or the one in Appendix B.

the top of the first column. This will allow you to track your sleep over the week and see any trends that emerge; for example, whether your sleep is different on weekends than it is on weekdays. (Your week of recording does not need to start with Monday, it can be any day of the week that you choose.)

Section on Sleep Timing

- **QUESTION 1**: Unless you are using a 24-hour clock system, make sure you put down A.M. or P.M. This will help you later when you are calculating how much time you spent in bed.

- **QUESTION 2**: This is the time between when you went to bed and when you turned out the lights, intending to go to sleep.

- **QUESTIONS 3, 4, and 5**: It is difficult to measure these things, so just provide your best estimates.

- **QUESTION 6**: This is the time from when you woke up in the morning until you got out of bed to start the day.

- **QUESTION 7**: As for Question 1, unless you are using a 24-hour clock system, specify A.M. or P.M.

Section on Sleep Quality

- For the *Quality of My Sleep*: Rate the overall quality of your sleep, from 1 to 10 where 1 = very poor and 10 = excellent.

Section on Naps, Alcohol, and Sleep Medication

- *Naps*: Specify the time and duration of any naps you had. This includes all naps, including ones that were unintended (e.g., you dozed off in front of the television).

- *Alcohol*: Specify time, type, and amount taken.

- *Sleep Medication*: Specify time, type, and amount taken. Include anything you took to try to sleep, including prescribed medication, herbal products, or something you bought at the drug store.

Feel free to use the space at the bottom of each column to record things that might have affected your sleep like headache, unusual medication, the days you were sick with a cold, a late night phone call that left you feeling stressed. If you think something may have affected your sleep, write it down.

At this point, it might be helpful for you to see what Julie did. So I will describe some aspects of her week and show you how she filled out her baseline sleep diary.

JULIE'S EXAMPLE

I saw Julie on a Tuesday and gave her the sleep diary form. She started filling in the first column that morning, and answered the questions about her previous night's sleep. The previous night was Monday, so she wrote "MON" at the top of the first column.

During the week that Julie was recording her first sleep diary, it was spring and the weather was fine, and work-related stress was low. Despite being relatively untroubled, Julie developed a headache on Monday evening. She went to bed at 8:30 P.M., thinking the headache would go away on its own, but she woke up in the night with a hot flash and the headache. After throwing off some blankets and trying not to disturb her husband, she took a headache medication (she jotted this down at the bottom of Monday's column). She had two more awakenings that night, and one of those happened with another hot flash. When she woke up for a third time, she felt cold and she pulled up her previously tossed blankets and went back to sleep. There were four other nights that she was aware of hot flashes.

On Tuesday night, she took half of a 7.5 mg tablet of zopiclone at 10:55 P.M. She took this because she was up late and wanted to make sure she got enough sleep prior to a meeting that was in her agenda for first thing the next morning. The zopiclone had been prescribed by her family doctor for occasional use. This helped Julie to fall asleep quite quickly that night.

On Wednesday, Julie had a phone call from her 23-year-old son that left her feeling somewhat stressed. When she woke up at 4:30 A.M., her mind went to her son's situation, what he had said, what she had said, what she wished she had said, and what she was planning to say next time she spoke to him. And then she wondered when she could speak with him next. She never did get back to sleep and got up at 6:00 anyway to get ready for work.

On Thursday evening, Julie went out with her husband to a fast food place and ate too much pepperoni pizza. She felt a bit nauseated when she went to bed at 9:00 and it took her a while to fall asleep. She took an over-the-counter nausea pill that night, hoping it would help her to doze off.

On Friday, Julie went to bed quite early—at 8:15 P.M.—because she was tired. You can see that she took about 45 minutes to fall asleep and she woke up twice, both times with hot flashes. The second time she woke up, she stayed awake for about 90 minutes before falling back asleep. During that 90 minutes, her mind was drifting around, including to thoughts about her work and about her son. She woke up at 5:00 A.M. and was unable to get back to sleep, even though it was the weekend and she would have liked more sleep.

On Saturday night, Julie relaxed with her husband and some friends at home. She had 3 glasses of wine over the evening. She went to bed later than usual, and fell asleep quite quickly, although she had several awakenings later in the night.

On Sunday afternoon, after spending 3 hours gardening, Julie lay down on the couch at about 4 P.M. and slept for an hour. You can see this was recorded as a nap. Later that evening, Julie felt the work week looming and she wanted to make sure to get enough sleep.

So she went to bed at 8:00 P.M. It took her about 2 hours to fall asleep. During this time, she was thinking about the work on her desk and planning how she would structure her day. She was also starting to feel anxious because the very thing that she was trying to get—enough sleep—was not happening.

You may think that Julie's sleep is better or worse than yours. That's okay. Everyone's different. Regardless of the severity of insomnia, the same sleep therapy techniques will work.

YOUR TURN

Now it's your turn. You can start right now. Take a minute, and think back to last night. What day of the week was it? Fill in the *DAY* at the top of the first column. Now you are on your way! Fill in the rest of the column if you can. If you can't remember last night's sleep, start the sleep diary tomorrow morning. After you have filled in the first column, place the sleep diary beside your bed or at the breakfast table so you will remember to record your information each morning for the rest of the week. Be patient with this process. In an attempt to move ahead with the baseline recording process, some people have tried to remember their entire previous week of sleep and have filled in the whole diary at one sitting. In doing so, they have usually missed details that turn out to be important later on. So even if you think you know your sleep patterns inside out, take one night at a time, and record your information. It is worth the investment of time. This process will allow you to really understand your current sleep patterns. Along the way, you may very well discover one or two things you hadn't noticed before.

BASELINE *(Julie) Sleep Diary for the week of:* April 19

DAY of the WEEK *Which night is being reported on?*	MON.	TUES
Sleep timing		
1. **I went to bed at** *(clock time):*	8:30 pm	11:30
2. **I turned out the lights after** *(minutes):*	15	0
3. **I fell asleep in** *(minutes):*	60	10
4. **I woke up ___ time(s) during the night.** *(number of awakenings):*	3 hot flashes	1
5. **The total duration of these awakenings was** *(minutes):*	75	90
6. **After awakening for the last time, I was in bed for** *(minutes):*	1	10
7. **I got up at** *(clock time):*	6:01 am	6:00 a
Sleep quality **The quality of my sleep was:** *1 = very poor; 10 = excellent*	4	6
Naps *Number, time and duration*	0	0
Alcohol *Time, amount, type*	/	/
Sleep Medication *Time, amount, type*	/	10:55p zopiclo 1/2 of 7.5
Notes:	headache – took pain medication early in the night	

WED.	THURS.	FRI.	SAT.	SUN.
:45 pm	9:00 pm	8:15 pm	11:15 pm	11:15 pm
0	15	15	0	20
45	60	45	5	120
0	1	2	4-5 hot flashes	3 hot flashes & washroom
0	90 hot flashes	95 hot flashes	25	70
90	10	130	135	3
OO am	6:00 am	7:00 am	7:15 am	6:03 am
4	4	4	5	3
0	0	0	0	1 at 4:00 pm for 60 mins
/	/	/	6-8pm 3 glasses of wine	5:00pm 1 glass of wine
/	8:50pm 1 Gravol	/	/	/
ke 4:30am view of a nversation	felt nauseated at bedtime	woke 5:00am	woke 5:00am	

BASELINE Sleep Diary for the week of: _____

DAY of the WEEK *Which night is being reported on?*		
Sleep timing		
1. **I went to bed at** *(clock time):*		
2. **I turned out the lights after** *(minutes):*		
3. **I fell asleep in** *(minutes):*		
4. **I woke up ___ time(s) during the night.** *(number of awakenings):*		
5. **The total duration of these awakenings was** *(minutes):*		
6. **After awakening for the last time, I was in bed for** *(minutes):*		
7. **I got up at** *(clock time):*		
Sleep quality — **The quality of my sleep was:** *1 = very poor; 10 = excellent*		
Naps *Number, time and duration*		
Alcohol *TIme, amount, type*		
Sleep Medication *TIme, amount, type*		
Notes:		

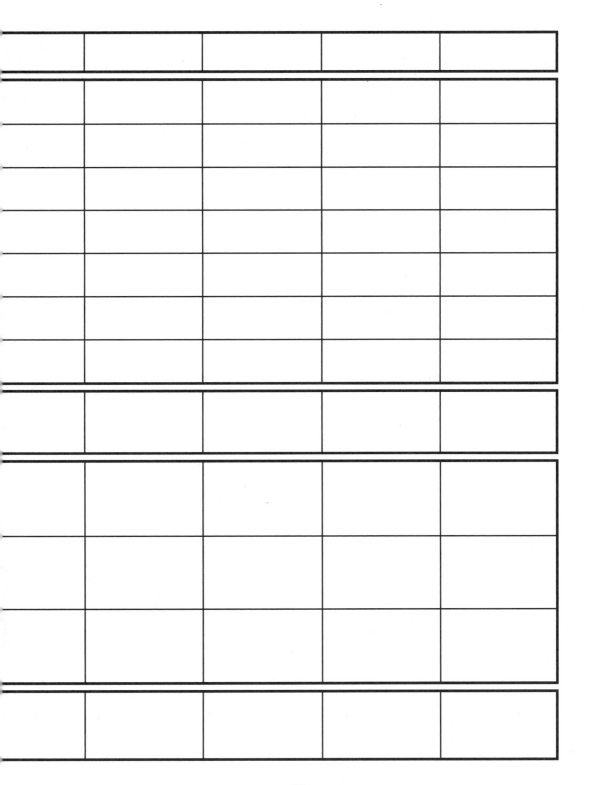

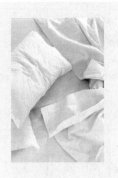

Chapter 7

What Type of Insomnia Do You Have?

Congratulations! You have a week's worth[1] of data about your sleep. Your completed sleep diaries will provide very interesting and useful information. Let's go through your baseline sleep diary and see what it tells you. You will be looking at certain rows of your sleep diary now, and other rows in the subsequent chapters. I will guide you through your sleep diary, pointing out what to look for. We will follow the same sequence that I use when I examine people's sleep diaries in the clinic, which is not necessarily the same order in which you filled out the sleep diary. Our first mission is to identify what type of insomnia you have.

On page 39 you will see a place to record what type(s) of insomnia you have. See the chart called "My Baseline Insomnia Types." You probably already have a sense of whether you have trouble initiating sleep (trouble falling asleep) or maintaining sleep (waking in the middle of the night or waking up too early) or both. However, let's take a closer look at some of your baseline sleep measures to confirm your specific insomnia type(s). This will also allow you to compare your baseline sleep to your sleep after Sleep Therapy.

INITIAL INSOMNIA

Read across your sleep diary at Question 3 and see how long it took you to fall asleep each night. Did it often (on 3 nights or more) take you longer than 30 minutes to fall asleep?

---

[1] I will talk about 7 nights of sleep diaries but if you collected 14 nights, you would do the same for all 14 nights.

If so, you are experiencing "initial insomnia."

Since Julie took a long time to get to sleep on 5 nights, she answered YES to this question.

3. I fell asleep in (minutes):	60	10	45	60	45	5	120

If you too answered yes, then circle "Initial Insomnia" in the right-hand column of the chart called "My Baseline Insomnia Types" on page 39.

MULTIPLE AWAKENINGS

Cast your eye across the diary at Question 4. Look at the number of awakenings you had each night. Did you often (on 3 nights or more) have more than 3 awakenings per night? If so, you can describe yourself as having "multiple awakenings." Julie answered this as NO because she had only one night with more than 3 awakenings.

4. I woke up ___ time(s) during the night. (number of awakenings):	3 hot flashes	1	0	1	2	4–5 hot flashes	3 hot flashes & washroom

If you often had more than 3 awakenings, then circle "multiple awakenings" in the right-hand column of the chart called "My Baseline Insomnia Types" on page 39.

MIDDLE INSOMNIA

Look at how long you were awake each night in Question 5. Is this number often (on 3 nights or more) greater than 30 minutes? If so, you are experiencing "middle insomnia." Julie answered YES to this question because 5 nights involved long awakenings.

5. The total duration of these awakenings was (minutes):	75	90	0	90 hot flashes	95 hot flashes	25	70

If you too had long awakenings on 3 nights or more, then circle "Middle Insomnia" in the chart called "My Baseline Insomnia Types" on page 39.

TERMINAL (END-OF-NIGHT) INSOMNIA

Look over the times that you were awake in bed in the morning at Question 6. Was this often (on 3 nights or more) 30 minutes or longer? If so, was this because you woke up earlier than you had wanted? If you are often waking up more than 30 minutes too early, then you can say you have "terminal" insomnia. If the word "terminal" sounds too ominous, feel free to call it "end-of-night" insomnia.

Note that terminal insomnia only applies to you if you are waking up earlier than you had intended. You can also have long times for Question 6 if you are lying around in bed in the morning after the alarm has gone off, or just relaxing in bed rather than getting up. Do *not* count such lying around times as terminal insomnia; just count the nights on which you woke up too early by more than 30 minutes.

Julie had 3 nights when she awakened much earlier than she had wanted to, so she answered YES.

6. After awakening for the last time, I was in bed for (minutes):	1	10	90	10	130	135	3

If you too answered yes, then circle "terminal insomnia" in the right-hand column of the chart called "My Baseline Insomnia Types" on page 39.

MORE THAN ONE TYPE

You have just looked at your baseline sleep diary for initial insomnia, multiple awakenings, middle insomnia, and terminal insomnia. It is quite common for people to have more than one type of insomnia problem. In the chart you may have circled several (up to 4) types; these are your insomnia types at baseline. Have a look at them. You will return to these categories later, after you have finished Sleep Therapy, to see if you still have any of these types of insomnia.

YOUR SLEEP QUALITY

Your impression of how you are sleeping is, of course, one of the most important measurements. In your sleep diary, the section in the middle of the form captures this information. Look across the days of the week, what are your "quality" ratings? Take your most common rating. If your scores are all over the map, calculate the average (by adding them up and dividing by 7). Julie's most common rating was 4.

The quality of my sleep was: 1 = very poor; 10 = excellent	4	6	4	4	4	5	3

Record your most common rating (or the average) in the chart on page 39 where it says "The quality of my sleep." This estimate of the quality of your baseline sleep will be very useful later on to compare with your future ratings as you proceed with Sleep Therapy.

MOVING ON

It is very, very useful to have a measure of your sleep at the starting point of the program. I hope this chapter has allowed you to identify your current insomnia type(s) and to rate your sleep quality. Next, you will be looking at several other aspects of your baseline sleep diary, and doing some arithmetic in order to obtain two values that will allow you to tailor the Sleep Therapy procedures specifically for you.

Julie's Baseline Insomnia Types:

What type of Insomnia do I have?	Circle all that apply
Long time to get to sleep (*more than 30 minutes*)	*Initial Insomnia* (circled)
Many awakenings (*more than 3*)	**Multiple Awakenings**
Long time awake during the night (*more than 30 minutes*)	*Middle Insomnia* (circled)
Waking up too early (*more than 30 minutes*)	*Terminal Insomnia* (circled)
The quality of my sleep	Most common rating: 4

My Baseline Insomnia Types:

What type of Insomnia do I have?	Circle all that apply
Long time to get to sleep (*more than 30 minutes*)	*Initial Insomnia*
Many awakenings (*more than 3*)	**Multiple Awakenings**
Long time awake during the night (*more than 30 minutes*)	**Middle Insomnia**
Waking up too early (*more than 30 minutes*)	**Terminal Insomnia** ✳
The quality of my sleep	Most common rating:

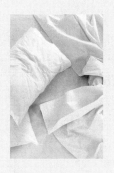

Chapter 8

Knowing Your Numbers

Two "nifty numbers" is what my friend Ryan calls them. By following the instructions in this chapter you will come up with two numbers that are essential for Sleep Therapy. As we saw in Chapter 5, Sleep Therapy is a combination of the most effective components of Cognitive Behavioral Therapy for Insomnia (CBT-I); it involves tailoring your bedtime and rise time for your sleep needs, and associating your bed with great sleep. Knowing your numbers will allow you to tailor your sleep improvement procedures for you and you alone. The first number is your "total sleep time," which is how much sleep you are getting now. The second number is your "sleep efficiency," which is how solid your sleep is.

You can use your baseline sleep diary to estimate fairly accurately your baseline values for total sleep time and sleep efficiency. So now's the time to find a calculator. You will be doing some straightforward arithmetic. (The calculations may look complicated but they are definitely easier and much faster than doing a page of your income tax return.) I will be showing you Julie's information so you can see how it's done. Don't expect to have the same or similar numbers as Julie did. Everyone is different.

YOUR BASELINE TOTAL SLEEP TIME

I will now show you how to estimate your baseline sleep duration, based on a night from your sleep diary. From your baseline sleep diary, choose a representative night—a night that you would consider to be an average night, not your worst or best night. Put a big asterisk or star at the top of that column so you can easily refer to it. Next, turn to the chart called "Calculating Your Baseline Total Sleep Time and Sleep Efficiency." You are going to take your

Calculating your Baseline Total Sleep Time and Sleep Efficiency

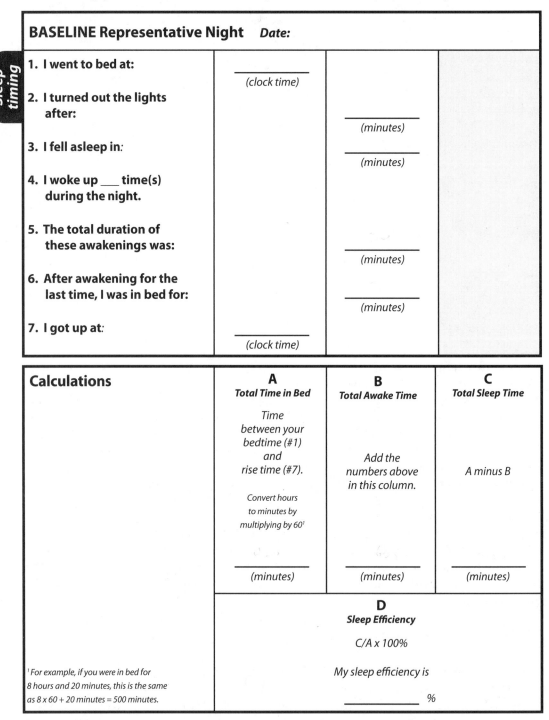

Sleep timing

BASELINE Representative Night   *Date:*

1. **I went to bed at:**

   _____
   (clock time)

2. **I turned out the lights after:**

   _____
   (minutes)

3. **I fell asleep in:**

   _____
   (minutes)

4. **I woke up ___ time(s) during the night.**

5. **The total duration of these awakenings was:**

   _____
   (minutes)

6. **After awakening for the last time, I was in bed for:**

   _____
   (minutes)

7. **I got up at:**

   _____
   (clock time)

Calculations

	A *Total Time in Bed*	**B** *Total Awake Time*	**C** *Total Sleep Time*
	Time between your bedtime (#1) and rise time (#7). *Convert hours to minutes by multiplying by 60*[1]	*Add the numbers above in this column.*	*A minus B*
	_____ *(minutes)*	_____ *(minutes)*	_____ *(minutes)*

D *Sleep Efficiency*
C/A x 100%
My sleep efficiency is _____ %

[1] *For example, if you were in bed for 8 hours and 20 minutes, this is the same as 8 x 60 + 20 minutes = 500 minutes.*

baseline representative night and copy the answers you had for Questions 1 to 7 onto the top part of this chart where you will find the same 7 questions. They are in the same order as on your sleep diary even though they are not all lined up vertically; you need to do a bit of zigzagging to enter the 7 numbers. This is merely to keep the clock times in one column and the minutes in another column.

Next, go the lower part of the chart where it says Calculations and sections A, B, and C. Here you will be coming up with your Total Sleep Time. This might look complicated, but all you will be doing is subtracting the number of minutes you were awake from the number of minutes you were in bed.

Start With Section A: Total Time in Bed

Total Time in Bed is the time between when you went to bed and when you got up in the morning. To determine this, look at the clock times you have entered in the column above A and figure out the difference. You will likely come up with the number of hours and minutes you were in bed. However, you need this number to be in minutes. So convert hours to minutes by multiplying by 60.

For example, if you were in bed for 9 hours and 20 minutes, this would be (9 hours × 60 minutes/hour) + 20 minutes = 560 minutes

Enter your Total Time in Bed on the appropriate line.

Now for Section B: Total Awake Time

For Total Awake Time, add up the times in the column above B. These are the durations you were awake during the night. Keep them in minutes. Put your answer for on the appropriate line.

For Section C: Total Sleep Time

For Total Sleep Time, take your answer for A and subtract your answer for B. This gives you your current amount of sleep in minutes. You will probably find it more meaningful to now express this in hours rather than minutes. So divide by 60. Then round to the nearest half-hour.

For example, if your Total Sleep Time is 370 minutes, this would be 370/60 = 6.1 hours. This rounds to 6.0 hours.

Other examples of rounding to the nearest half hour: If you had 5.7 hours, this rounds to 5.5 hours. If you had 5.8 hours, this rounds to 6.0 hours.

Now you have the number of hours, to the nearest half hour, that you are sleeping at baseline. Put this value in the box at the top of the next page for safekeeping. You will be using it when you begin Sleep Therapy.

My Baseline Total Sleep Time (in hours, to the nearest half hour):

6

If these calculations seem daunting, follow Julie's example first (near the end of this chapter) and then do the calculations for your own representative night. Note that you will be using minutes as units until you get to the last step when you will convert minutes into hours.

YOUR BASELINE SLEEP EFFICIENCY

Sleep efficiency is a measure of how solid your sleep is. It is the percentage of the time that you were asleep while in bed. Let's say that last night I collapsed into bed, immediately fell asleep, slept without interruption, and then leapt out of bed as soon as I woke up this morning. I would have a sleep efficiency of 100%. In contrast, if I didn't sleep at all—not even for 1 minute—I would have a sleep efficiency of 0%. Neither of these extremes is typical in real life, although sleep efficiencies can get very high and very low. To give you a feel for different sleep efficiency levels, a sleep efficiency of 30% is very low, a sleep efficiency of 60% is low, a sleep efficiency of 85% is quite high, and a sleep efficiency of 95% is very high.

Proceed to section D on the chart to calculate your Baseline Sleep Efficiency. You take your Total Sleep Time (C, in minutes) and divide it by your Total Time in Bed (A, in minutes). Then multiply by 100 to get the percentage. This is your Baseline Sleep Efficiency. Place this value in the box below. If you would like an example, have a look at Julie's calculations.

My Baseline Sleep Efficiency: _____%

You will be able to compare your Baseline Sleep Efficiency with your future sleep efficiencies. Also, in upcoming chapters you will see how to use your sleep efficiency values over time to direct your Sleep Therapy.

JULIE'S BASELINE TOTAL SLEEP TIME

Julie chose Thursday, April 22, as a representative night of her baseline week. She looked at the Sleep Timing section of her sleep diary for that night and copied her answers to Questions 1 to 7 into the chart called Julie's Baseline Total Sleep Time and Sleep Efficiency. You will notice that the clock times are in the first column and the durations are in the second column of the new chart, in the exact same order as on the sleep diary.

For Section A: Total Time in Bed

Julie computed the time between 9:00 p.m. and 6:00 a.m. She was in bed for a total of 9 hours. She converted this to minutes (multiplied by 60), to get 540 minutes.

For Section B: Total Awake Time

Julie summed the durations in the column above B; that is, she added up all the time she was awake during the night. She got 175 minutes.

For Section C: Total Sleep Time

Julie took her Total Time in Bed (540 minutes) and subtracted her Total Awake Time (175) and got 365 minutes. To convert this to hours, she divided by 60 and got 6.08 hours. She then rounded this to the nearest half hour and got 6.0 hours. So her Baseline Total Sleep Time was 6.0 hours. She put this in the box below.

Julie's Baseline Total Sleep Time (in hours, to the nearest half hour):

_6.0_

JULIE'S SLEEP EFFICIENCY

Julie went to section D. She divided her Total Sleep Time at C (in minutes) by her Total Time in Bed at A (in minutes). This was 365 divided by 540. She then multiplied by 100%. This gave her 68%. This was her Baseline Sleep Efficiency. She put this in the box below.

Julie's Baseline Sleep Efficiency: _68_ %

Julie's Baseline Total Sleep Time and Sleep Efficiency

BASELINE Representative Night		Date: Thurs Apr 22	
1. I went to bed at:	9:00pm *(clock time)*		
2. I turned out the lights after:		15 *(minutes)*	
3. I fell asleep in:		60 *(minutes)*	
4. I woke up __1__ time(s) during the night.			
5. The total duration of these awakenings was:		90 *(minutes)*	
6. After awakening for the last time, I was in bed for:		10 *(minutes)*	
7. I got up at:	6:00am *(clock time)*		

Sleep timing

Calculations	**A** Total Time in Bed	**B** Total Awake Time	**C** Total Sleep Time
	Time between your bedtime (#1) and rise time (#7). Convert hours to minutes by multiplying by 60[1]	Add the numbers above in this column.	A minus B
9 hrs = (9x60) = 540 mins	540 *(minutes)*	175 *(minutes)*	365 *(minutes)*

	D Sleep Efficiency C/A x 100%
[1] For example, if you were in bed for 8 hours and 20 minutes, this is the same as 8 x 60 + 20 minutes = 500 minutes.	My sleep efficiency is __68__ %

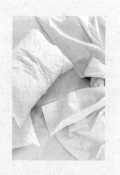

Chapter 9

Things to Take Care of Right Away

Now that you have established the nature of your insomnia in Chapter 7 and you know your numbers from Chapter 8, it's time to check a few other things. These are things over which you have direct control. So, if they are out-of-whack and are creating poor sleep, they can be addressed right away. You will now be perusing your sleep diary for three things: naps, alcohol, and sleep medication. Not that any of these things is bad (they are often very good), you just want to make sure that they are not interfering with your nighttime sleep. If they are interfering, it is much easier to deal with them now, before you go further.

Some of you will breeze right through this chapter because you don't take naps, you don't drink alcohol, and/or you don't take any sleep medication. Many others will discover that your nap patterns are fine, or that your alcohol consumption or sleeping medication use are no problem. A few of you will find that there is something you can adjust now to start improving your sleep right away. In any event, you will find it helpful to carefully check these things.

YOUR NAPS

Look across your baseline sleep diary and see on how many days you napped. Some people never nap; if this is you, you can skip this section. If you did nap, were your naps inadvertent or intentional? If they were *inadvertent* (you fell asleep in front of the television, or you fell asleep after breakfast, or at your desk), and you had several of these sleeps during the week, this can be a sign of "excessive daytime sleepiness." Sometimes this happens when you are cutting short your sleep time due to work, family, or other demands. For example, if you are working at three jobs and you only have 4 hours available for sleep, or if you are staying up late to drive the kids around and then getting up at 4:00 a.m. to get more things done before everyone else gets up, then you are cutting short your time for sleep. This results in a sleep deficit that may cause you to be very sleepy and to fall asleep in various situations during the day. This is a fixable situation: You need to make sleep a priority and allow enough time for it.

If you are not cutting short your sleep to do things, then your sleepiness and inadvertent naps are more likely related to a medical condition, a substance or medication you are taking, or a sleep disorder *other* than insomnia. Usually this type of excessive sleepiness does *not* occur with insomnia unless something else is causing it. To get help sorting out what is causing the daytime sleepiness, I recommend that you visit your family doctor to look into the source of the sleepiness and how to reduce or manage it.

If your naps were *intentional* (e.g., you lay down for a nap on Sunday afternoon), then look at the timing of each nap.

What time of day do you take your naps? _____

Did you know that 1:00 pm to 4:00 p.m. is the prime napping zone? We humans are predisposed to nap in the afternoon. Several lines of evidence point to this. Mid-afternoon corresponds to nap time in many siesta cultures, the most frequent nap time of young children before they "grow out of" napping, and the most popular nap time for adults of all ages. There are physical signs, too, that an afternoon nap is normal and natural. For example, in the early afternoon, we experience the so-called "post-lunch dip," which is a dip in alertness and work performance. Unrelated to food, it seems instead to be a natural time to drift off to sleep. There is also a subtle, transient drop in our body temperature at this time, indicating that our body is readying itself for sleep. The mid-afternoon is the time when people fall asleep most quickly during the day if given the opportunity in a sleep lab. As if you needed more rationale to take a nap in this zone, naps at this time are rich in restorative deep sleep. (Naps in the morning tend to have more REM, the stage in which most of our dreaming occurs; see Appendix A for information about sleep stages.) Furthermore, naps in this zone are unlikely to interfere with your nighttime sleep. We know this from studies of naps and subsequent sleep. So, in general, for people who have regular nighttime sleeping hours, the zone 1:00–4:00 p.m. appears to be the best time to take a nap. If your naps are earlier or later than this, consider moving them into the prime nap zone.

Now, have a look at the duration of each nap. How long was it? I recommend limiting your nap to 1 hour or less. This is so you build up sufficient biological sleep drive for your nighttime sleep. The sleep drive is, in some ways, like the eating drive or hunger. You don't want to have a big meal in the afternoon if you are planning to have a banquet in the evening. You will want to have a snack instead, so that your hunger has built up by the evening, allowing you to enjoy the banquet.

To sum up, you will achieve your best sleep by limiting your nap to 1 hour or less in duration, within the 1:00–4:00 p.m. zone. If you are already doing this, then congratulations; you are a fabulous napper!

Naps *Number, time, and duration*	○	○	○	○	○	○	1 at 4:00pm for 60 mins

Julie had an afternoon nap on Sunday but it started at about 4:00 p.m. which was a bit late. She decided to pay attention to her nap timing for the next week and to lie down by 3:00 p.m. so she would be up by 4:00 p.m.

ALCOHOL

If you don't use alcohol, just skip this section. If you do enjoy a drink of any type of alcohol, take a look at your Baseline Sleep Diary and see on how many days you had alcohol, at what time, and what amount. Alcohol in low doses (e.g., one standard drink[1]) sometimes helps us to fall asleep quickly. However, alcohol disrupts sleep significantly later in the night; it leads to lighter sleep and more awakenings. All sleep stages are affected by alcohol but the most obvious effects are on stage REM (dream sleep). This stage is abnormally suppressed during the first part of the night, and it then "rebounds"—occurs with a vengeance—in the latter part of the night as the blood alcohol level drops to zero. Along with the REM rebound, there is sleep disruption, more dreaming, and sometimes an alarming state with nightmares, increased heart rate, and sweating. The more alcohol we consume, the greater the sleep disruption. The amount of sleep disruption also depends on many other factors like the exact timing of the drink(s), how much food was eaten with the alcohol, body size, weight, gender, age, liver health, genetic factors, and past patterns of alcohol use.

Given all these factors that go into predicting the effect of alcohol on sleep, it is difficult to give exact recommendations about the quantity and timing of drinking that will minimize effects on sleep. *Basically, less is better, and earlier is better.* A common recommendation is to not drink within 4 to 6 hours of bedtime. This is roughly the amount of time for a young man to absorb and metabolize 2 standard drinks, taken without food, so that the alcohol is no longer in the blood. This is just a rough guide. Alcohol can exert effects on sleep even after it is no longer in the bloodstream. One study had 61-year-old men drinking 3 standard drinks at "happy hour" before dinner, 6 hours before bed. The researchers confirmed that the alcohol was no longer in their system at bedtime. Their sleep that night was compared to a control night with a non alcoholic happy hour. Sleep on the alcoholic happy

---

[1] One standard drink is 5 oz. of wine (12% alcohol), 1.5 oz. of spirits (40% alcohol), or 12 oz. of beer (5% alcohol).

hour night was broken up, the sleep stages were altered (REM was suppressed), and there was more wakefulness in the second half of the night. All this happened, even though all the alcohol had cleared out of their blood before they went to bed! Essentially, alcohol interferes with the quality, quantity, and sleep stage composition of sleep, and these effects can last for many hours—well into the night and the next morning.

Look at the nights with alcohol and without. Are there differences in those nights? Are they better, worse, or the same with alcohol? Based on what you discover, you may decide to do nothing at all, or you may decide to alter the timing or the amount of alcohol.

If you had a drink each night, it will of course be difficult to compare with no-alcohol nights. If this is part of your lifestyle, then your body is accustomed to this pattern of alcohol intake. Someone who had wine with dinner every night asked me if she should keep sleep diaries for a usual week and then for another week without alcohol. I don't recommend this. This is because your sleep will probably be more disturbed without the usual alcohol because your sleep system has become accustomed to having the alcohol on board. Taking it away may lead to a temporary worsening of sleep. If you are okay with your current pattern of alcohol use, and it is not more than 1–2 drinks, taken at least 4 to 6 hours before sleep, then you are probably fine in terms of effects on your sleep.

In addition to effects on your sleep, other aspects of health can be affected by alcohol. At certain levels, alcohol use increases the risk of cardiovascular disease (increased chance of heart attack and stroke), cancer, liver disease, accidents and falls, and mental health problems. If you wonder whether alcohol is affecting your health, information is available to help you estimate your health risk. Contact your public health unit or check the Low Risk Drinking Guidelines www.lrdg.net or the National Institute on Alcohol Abuse and Alcoholism website www.niaaa.nih.gov.

Alcohol Time, amount, type	/	/	/	/	/	6–8pm 3 glasses of wine	5:00pm 1 glass of wine

Julie had wine on Saturday and Sunday evenings. Looking at her baseline sleep diary, she noticed that after her 3 glasses of wine on Saturday night she fell asleep quickly, but later in the night she had 4–5 brief awakenings. Julie decided she would drink fewer than 3 glasses of wine in case that was affecting her sleep. Make your own observations. Now's your chance to change the amount or timing of your beer or wine or cocktail depending on what you see in this baseline diary.

SLEEP MEDICATION

If you are not taking any substances to help you sleep you can skip this section. Are you taking a prescribed sleep medication? Are you taking an over-the-counter sleep remedy? If so, please read more about the various sleep medications in Chapter 22. In general, if you have been taking benzodiazepines (such as lorazepam, clonazepam, oxazepam, temazepam, etc.) or "z-drugs" (such as zopiclone or zolpidem) every night for more than 1 month, and especially if you are not happy with your sleep, then you may want to talk to your family physician about a slow withdrawal from this medication. A very slow schedule is necessary to prevent "rebound insomnia," which is a worsening of your insomnia.

Make sure you continue to track your use of these medications to see if your use goes down with Sleep Therapy. Most people who take these medications on an occasional basis find they need them less and less as they proceed with Sleep Therapy. If you do use sleep medications, it is important to take them only at or before your bedtime, and not in the middle of the night (unless of course they are designed to be used in the middle of the night, like zaleplon). If taken later than your bedtime they may cause you to have a hard time waking up in the morning, and to feel groggy. This is because the medication has not had adequate time to leave your bloodstream, and is still affecting your central nervous system. For other situations of taking medication, over-the-counter aids, or herbal products, please read the relevant sections of Chapter 22 for further information.

Sleep Medication *Time, amount, type*		10:55pm zopi- clone 1/2 of 7.5mg		8:50pm 1 Gra- vol			
	/		/		/	/	/

Julie took a sleeping pill on one night of her baseline week. She uses it occasionally. It seemed to help her fall asleep and on that night she had a pretty good sleep despite a long awakening during the night. She used an anti-nausea medication on another night, hoping that it would also help her to fall asleep.

SLEEP MEDICATION AND ALCOHOL

If you are taking sleep medication, it can be dangerous to also drink alcohol. Both substances relax the nervous system, leading to reduced alertness, and slowed, shallow breathing. The combined effect can be hazardous and even lethal. So if you take sleep medication, make sure to avoid alcohol that day and night. And read the instructions on the medication label about alcohol use.

Solving Your Insomnia

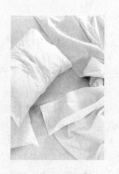

Chapter 10

The Essential Elements of
Sleep Therapy

Two essential elements form Sleep Therapy. In this chapter, I will explain these elements, which are based on sleep science and psychology principles. Many people find this background intriguing. What's more, it is always easier to carry out techniques when you understand how they work. The elements of Sleep Therapy are: a) uncovering your natural sleep processes, and b) associating your bed with sleep.

UNCOVERING YOUR NATURAL SLEEP PROCESSES

By understanding how sleep comes and goes in the natural state we can see more clearly how to sleep well. It is by allowing these sleep processes to operate without interference that we can experience good sleep. Let's start by looking at two very important biological processes that regulate sleep and wakefulness.[1]

---

[1] In 1982, Dr. Alexander Borbély of Switzerland proposed a model of sleep regulation. It was called the Two-Process Model. Several other models have been proposed since then, some being more sophisticated variations or refinements, but most of them still rest on the assumption that there are two main processes. The Two-Process Model has been extremely useful in understanding our sleep and predicting the timing of our best sleep.

Sleep's Homeostatic Process

Homeostatic processes are mechanisms in our bodies that maintain a state of equilibrium. For example, homeostatic processes control and balance the level of glucose in our blood, the water content in our tissues, and regulate our temperature, heart rate, and blood pressure. Likewise, we have a homeostatic mechanism that regulates our propensity to sleep. Basically the longer we stay awake, the more likely we are to fall asleep and to stay asleep. This phenomenon is evident in toddlers when they are up past their regular bedtime—they may just fall asleep wherever they are. The parents have to cart them off to bed. The toddler's deep and undisturbed sleep is the homeostatic sleep process at work. You, too, will be staying up past your usual bedtime in order to achieve good sleep. Shortly, I will guide you through the calculation of exactly how late you will need to stay up in order to start having your homeostatic sleep process working for you.

Sleep's Circadian Process

The second process is a circadian rhythm. The word circadian comes from Latin: *circa* = about, around; and *diem* = a day. These are rhythms that go through one cycle approximately every 24 hours. Why 24 hours? Because one light-dark cycle on Earth is 24 hours long, and like other species, we are well adapted to the rotation rate of our planet. These internal rhythms are so strong that they persist even if we are in a cave without light-dark information. They are controlled by an internal clock in a part of the brain called the suprachiasmatic nucleus of the hypothalamus. Several of our hormones have a circadian pattern of release, as do aspects of our heart function, kidney function, and immune system. Did you know that every 24 hours our body temperature rises and falls in a predictable way? This circadian fluctuation is quite small (up to about 1 degree C entigrade) but is very reliable. Our sleep propensity has a circadian rhythm and it is linked to our temperature rhythm: We are most likely to fall asleep as our body temperature is declining in the evening and most likely to wake up as our body temperature is rising in the morning. Every 24 hours there is a "prime time" to fall asleep. This period is when you are likely to fall asleep quickly and stay asleep for the night. I will be showing you how to stabilize and strengthen your circadian rhythm of sleep-wakefulness in order to obtain optimal sleep.

We Can Use These Processes to Sleep Well

The techniques that you will learn in this section are all about becoming familiar with your own sleep processes, removing interference with them, and strengthening them in order to maximize the chances of good, sound sleep. Remember that we do not achieve sleep by actively searching for it. Rather, we do things to optimize the conditions for good sleep and that's all. We leave the rest to our internal sleep processes. I will now explain the specific techniques that reverse insomnia, and you will see how your homeostatic and circadian sleep processes can work for you.

Stay Up Late

Staying up late allows our homeostatic sleep mechanisms to shift into gear. You will be figuring out how late you need to stay up to get your homeostatic process working for you. We will use a technique called "sleep restriction."[2] Years of research and clinical experience have shown sleep restriction to be a top treatment for insomnia. Sleep restriction is actually about restricting your *time in bed*. You will set a "bedtime" and "threshold rise time" that will limit your time in bed. You will use information from your sleep diaries to determine these times. As your sleep improves, you will adjust your bedtime from week to week.

Setting your "threshold" bedtime and rise time for the first week of Sleep Therapy

To determine these times, follow the instructions in the next table. Julie's table is shown as an example.

Julie's threshold bedtime and rise time

Pick your threshold rise time Pick a rise time that you can maintain 7 days per week. It needs to work for you and, of course, be early enough to allow you to get to work, or start your activities on time.	*a.* 6:00am This is your **threshold rise time**
Recall your total sleep time Take your total sleep time in hours (to the nearest half hour) that you calculated in Chapter 8, pages 43–44.	*b.* 6.0 hrs If this number is less than 5.0 hours, then replace it with 5.0.
Calculate your threshold bedtime Take your threshold rise time (a) and subtract (i.e., go backwards around the clock) your total sleep time (b).	*c.* *a - b =* midnight This is your **threshold bed time** for the first week
Julie's **threshold bedtime** *and* **threshold rise time**. **Bedtime:** midnight **Rise Time:** 6:00am	

---

[2] This technique was described in 1987 by Dr. A. J. Spielman and colleagues.

My threshold bedtime and rise time

Pick your threshold rise time Pick a rise time that you can maintain 7 days per week. It needs to work for you and, of course, be early enough to allow you to get to work, or start your activities on time.	**a.** _____ This is your **threshold rise time**
Recall your total sleep time Take your total sleep time in hours (to the nearest half hour) that you calculated in Chapter 8, pages 43–44.	**b.** _____ hrs If this number is less than 5.0 hours, then replace it with 5.0.
Calculate your threshold bedtime Take your threshold rise time (a) and subtract (i.e., go backwards around the clock) your total sleep time (b).	**c.** $a - b =$ _____ This is your **threshold bed time** for the first week
Enter your **threshold bedtime** and **threshold rise time** below. **Bedtime:** _____ **Rise Time:** _____	

Perhaps your threshold bedtime seems extremely late to you. People in our program sometimes drop their jaw in disbelief at having to stay up until 1:00 or 3:00 a.m. or whatever their threshold bedtime is for the first week. However, remember that this is just for a short time (the first week) to build up your homeostatic sleep process. It *should* seem a bit extreme. Think of that toddler who konks out after being up too late. You, too, will be staying up much too late. You will do this for a few days in order to allow your sleep to become solid, so you are sleeping like a log. You will be adjusting your bedtime, usually earlier, week by week. I will be showing you how to adjust your bedtime after the first week of Sleep Therapy.

How will you stay up until the late hour that is your threshold bedtime? You can use your imagination now to think of what you will be doing with that extra time. Maybe there is a project you have wanted to do and never "got around to it." Maybe you want to embark on something totally new like reading a book on how to identify the various fir trees, or learning a new art form. Maybe you just want to fold some laundry or watch a late-night TV show. Maybe you want to write an old-fashioned letter to your aunt. You will now have some extra hours in the week to work with. Start planning your nighttime activities now for the first week of Sleep Therapy!

Get Up at the Same Time Every Day

If you already get up around the same time 7 days a week, good for you. This part will be simple for you and you are already helping your circadian sleep process. If you have rise times that change from day to day, your task is clear. You will need to get up and out of bed at your threshold rise time each morning of Sleep Therapy. Why? Having a set rise time,

7 days a week is an excellent way of "entraining" (strengthening and anchoring) your circadian sleep process. When this rhythm is strong, you will be more likely to sleep well. It will allow you to consistently become sleepy in the evening as your body temperature falls, for you to sleep well overnight as your body temperature reaches its trough, and for you to wake up as your body temperature rises in the morning.

Will getting up at the same time every day be difficult for you? Only if you love sleeping in late on weekends or days off. People who have to give up their sleep-ins sometimes find it helpful to think of the things they can do with the extra time in the morning. One person used it as an opportunity to enjoy the bird activity in her yard. You can drum up reasons for getting up. If it really is painful for you to get up at the same time every day of the week, you can think of it as short-term pain for longer-term gain. You will not have to do this for the rest of your life (unless you want to). You are using this procedure at this time to strengthen your circadian sleep process in order to optimize your sleep. Also, it might help to know that you don't have to wake up at *precisely* the same time each morning, 15 minutes earlier or later is usually okay.

ASSOCIATING YOUR BED WITH SLEEP

This element of Sleep Therapy is based on something called "conditioning" or "learned associations." These are connections we make in our mind (automatically) between two things that occur together on several occasions. For example, some people find that when they go home at the end of the day and enter their kitchen, they immediately feel like eating—even if they are not truly hungry—because they have come to associate that time of day and their kitchen with eating. You may have heard of Pavlov's dogs who started to salivate whenever a bell rang, after the bell had been paired with food several times. In the case of sleep, you want to learn to *associate your bed with sleep*.

Your Bed Is for Sleep

When we have insomnia, our bed becomes associated with sleeplessness and the frustration that accompanies it. We can reverse this by starting to pair our bed with sleep and sleep alone, sexual activity being the only exception. The best way to do this is by following some basic instructions called "Stimulus Control Therapy."[3] This technique has been tested in many research facilities and clinics and is one of the most effective treatments for insomnia. I will now outline and explain the basic instructions for associating your bed with sleep.

Something that happens to many people with insomnia is that they drift to another bed, or to the couch, in order to get better sleep. Sometimes this leads to good sleep in the new location, but it doesn't help you to sleep well in your own bed. I recommend that you choose the bed that is the one you want to sleep well in, and use only that bed. This is the place you will be associating with good sleep. The following strategies will allow you to associate your bed with sleep and sleepiness.

---

[3] Stimulus control therapy was originally developed by Dr. Richard Bootzin, who presented the technique at a conference in 1972.

Go to bed only when sleepy and not before your threshold bedtime

A key word here is "sleepy." Do you know how sleepy feels? Sometimes we forget what the physical signs of sleepiness are. For some people sleepiness is experienced as yawning. Other possible signs are blurring eyesight and losing visual focus. For example, you might notice a blurring of the lines in a book you are reading. You lose concentration on what you are doing: You may find yourself reading a sentence or paragraph over and over again because you lost track. Your head may nod. You may feel like dozing off. The idea is not to go to bed until you feel some of the physical signs of sleepiness. This is because you want to associate your bed and bedroom with sleepiness and sleep.

You may be wondering if sleepiness is the same thing as being tired or fatigued. In day-to-day conversation, people often use these words interchangeably. However, as a sleep researcher, I am careful to distinguish these words. "Sleepiness" is the tendency to sleep. "Fatigue" is a physical or mental exhaustion that often comes from exertion. "Tiredness" is weariness, like fatigue. Sometimes we feel drained, mentally or physically, and fatigued and tired, yet we are not sleepy. For this particular technique, it is important that you do not go to bed before you are actually *sleepy*.

So you go to bed when sleepy and *not before your threshold bedtime*. What is this bedtime? This is the threshold bedtime that you have just set for yourself for the initial week. So, you will need to stay up at least until the threshold bedtime and then only go to bed if you are also sleepy. If it is your threshold bedtime and you are not sleepy, then stay up until you are sleepy.

Use the bed only for sleeping

Sexual activity is the only exception. Do not watch television, listen to the radio, use electronic devices, eat, or read in bed. This strategy is designed to help you associate your bed with sleep and not other miscellaneous things. Forbidden electronic devices include MP3 players, iPods, computers of any type, cell phones, e-book readers, and so on. If these are in the bedroom, they will not help your sleep. Remove them! If you use the alarm on your cell phone to wake you in the morning, then find an old-fashioned alarm clock to use instead. Turn off the cell phone and put it away, preferably in another room.

Get Out of Bed When You Are Not Sleeping

Part of strengthening the association of your bed with sleep is to make sure that your bed is *not* associated with being awake. So you need to be out of bed when you are not sleeping.

Leave the bed if you can't fall asleep or go back to sleep within 10–15 minutes

Return when sleepy. Repeat this step as often as necessary during the night. This helps you associate your bed with sleep, rather than wakefulness. Therefore, if you are awake for longer than 10-15 minutes, leave the bed. You do not need to, and you shouldn't, watch the clock. The 10-15 minutes is a rough guideline. When you find yourself awake in bed after a few minutes, leave the bed.

Go to another room and do something low-key and pleasant. You may decide to watch television. This may be stimulating rather than relaxing, depending on the program. If so, choose another less-stimulating activity. It is best to avoid the computer because the light from the screen can be alerting. Many people read a book, magazine, or newspaper. Don't sit under a very bright light. Use a light that is bright enough to read comfortably, but not the brightest one in the house. Others do jigsaw puzzles, crosswords, or play solitaire with a deck of cards. Some people do household things, like folding laundry; I used to wash dishes. Carry on your activity until you experience physical signs of sleepiness and then return to bed. If you are then awake in bed again for more than 15 minutes, don't get discouraged, just get up again and repeat the same steps.

It is much easier to get out of bed in the night if you prepare yourself for this possibility. If it is cold, lay a housecoat or big sweater and your woolly slippers next to your bed so that you will be warm enough when you are out of bed. A basket with the things you will need during your wake episodes can help reduce decision making during the night. Simply grab your basket, go to another room and start your activity.

What about other members of the household? Of course, you will go about your nighttime activity quietly so as not to disturb others' sleep. You may want to let certain people, like your bed partner, know what you are doing so that they understand. You can say that you are following instructions about going to bed and getting out of bed as part of a program to improve your sleep. You can tell them not to worry about you if they notice you coming and going from the bedroom.

Get out of bed when you wake up in the morning

No lounging around in bed after you wake up in the morning! The reason you want to get up right away is that you do *not* want to associate your bed with being awake. It is important to not spend extra time in bed. Some people find it very difficult to get moving out of bed after they wake up, especially on weekends. It is pleasant to lie there, warm and comfy. However, for the good of your future sleep, try to roll out of bed within 5 minutes, and start your day. Think of something to get up for—a cup of coffee or tea perhaps, or a bath, a stroll down the street, a flip through the newspaper.

PUTTING THE ELEMENTS INTO ACTION

Now that you know the essential elements and the basic strategies of Sleep Therapy, you are well prepared to put Sleep Therapy into action.

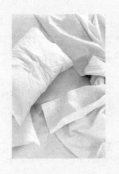

Chapter 11

Starting Sleep Therapy

Here's where you put all of this knowledge together and move right along to better sleep! You will be using the elements outlined in the previous chapter to start sleeping well. I have summarized the strategies of Sleep Therapy in 6 specific steps. The first 4 steps are based directly on what you have just read in Chapter 10. Carefully go over these first 4 instructions now to be sure of them. Fill in your initial threshold bedtime at step 1 and your initial threshold rise time at step 2. The last 2 steps are additional strategies to support your progress with Sleep Therapy. Specifically, if the procedures make you very sleepy, there is an option to have an afternoon nap (step 5); and you will be tracking your sleep with a sleep diary (step 6).

The steps of Sleep Therapy appear to be simple, but they require some time and effort. The effects may not be immediate, but if you follow them closely, after a few nights of practice, benefits will be evident. Do not get discouraged if you initially have some disrupted nights. The most important factor that determines whether your sleep will improve or not is the consistency with which you follow the steps.

Six Steps to Solid Sleep

1. Go to bed only when sleepy and not before your threshold bedtime. _____
   Fill in the threshold bedtime that you set in Chapter 10 (pages 57–58).

2. Maintain a regular threshold rise time in the morning. _____
   Fill in the threshold rise time that you chose in Chapter 10 (pages 57–58).

3. Use the bed only for sleeping. Sexual activity is the only exception. Do not watch television, listen to the radio, use electronic devices, eat, or read in bed.

4. Leave the bed if you can't fall asleep or go back to sleep within 10–15 minutes. Return when sleepy. Repeat this step as often as necessary during the night.

5. If sleepiness is overwhelming, you may take a short nap (no longer than 1 hour) in the afternoon, starting before 3 p.m.

6. Maintain a sleep diary.

Some Words About Steps 5 and 6

If sleepiness is overwhelming, you may take a short nap (no longer than 1 hour) in the afternoon, starting before 3 p.m.

Because you may be very sleepy during the day, especially when you first start this schedule, this is an optional step that may come in handy. Many programs recommend that you avoid daytime naps entirely because naps may make it harder to sleep at night. While this is partially true, we also know that humans are biologically predisposed to have a nap in the afternoon if circumstances permit. A nap (shorter than 1 hour in duration) taken in the afternoon, starting before 3 p.m. is unlikely to negatively affect your nighttime sleep. You *do* want to avoid multiple naps and naps that occur at times other than the "prime nap zone." (The rationale for the timing of a nap is found in Chapter 9.) So, if you are having a hard time with the initial sleep deprivation that occurs with the first 2 steps of Sleep Therapy, you can always take a brief nap. If you are working at a day job, then it may not be possible to do so in that period. Many places do not yet appreciate the benefits of napping at work! If that's the case, you may have to use your nap option on your days off.

Maintain a sleep diary

Keeping a sleep diary will show you right away how your sleep improves as a result of your actions. So track your progress by filling in a column of a sleep diary each morning.

You Should Know

- Following the first two instructions may involve a degree of short-term sleep deprivation; therefore you should be prepared for this. Some people choose to start it on a weekend so that most of the sleep deprivation will occur when they don't need to be performing brilliantly.

- Start this schedule of going to bed and getting up from bed when you have an excellent chance of following it carefully. If you are just about to travel to another time zone, now is not the time to begin the six steps. Wait until you are settled back in your normal house, bed, and time zone.

- If work or home life is just too busy and stressful to be able to follow this plan closely, you may want to delay using this approach until it fits into your days and nights in a more manageable way.

- You may want to explain what you are doing to your family members, especially the person who shares your bed. Help them understand that you may have odd bedtimes and rise times for a while, but this is a temporary strategy to improve your sleep. Elicit their moral support!

- If you find that you are very sleepy during this program (especially likely in the first few days), be sure to avoid driving and other potentially dangerous activities that require vigilance during this time.

WEEK 1

So, now that you have your 6 steps to solid sleep in front of you with your threshold bedtime and rise time for the first week, here's what you do. Follow these 6 instructions for a week. Remember, you can go to bed later than, but not earlier than, your threshold bedtime. Recall that you also need to be sleepy before going to bed. You can get up earlier than, but not later than, the threshold rise time. You need to keep track of each night's sleep with a sleep diary—this is very important. Use the sleep diary (Week 1) at the end of this chapter. Make sure to put in the start date and your initial threshold bedtime and rise time at the top.

You may be tired and sleepy and somewhat miserable for a few days. Hang in there, it will get much better! A typical pattern that people encounter is some sleep deprivation for the first 3-4 days and then their sleep improves markedly and they feel better. Using these techniques takes some perseverance. But know that it is worth it. Be kind to yourself and have faith that you are using the most effective strategies we have to reverse insomnia, and don't think about it too much!

WEEK 1 Sleep Diary for the week of: _____

DAY of the WEEK *Which night is being reported on?*		
1. I went to bed at *(clock time):*		
2. I turned out the lights after *(minutes):*		
3. I fell asleep in *(minutes):*		
4. I woke up ___ time(s) during the night. *(number of awakenings):*		
5. The total duration of these awakenings was *(minutes):*		
6. After awakening for the last time, I was in bed for *(minutes):*		
7. I got up at *(clock time):*		
The quality of my sleep was: *1 = very poor; 10 = excellent*		
Naps *Number, time and duration*		
Alcohol *TIme, amount, type*		
Sleep Medication *TIme, amount, type*		
Notes:		

Sleep timing (rows 1–7)

Sleep quality (quality row)

Bedtime: _____ **Rise Time:** _____

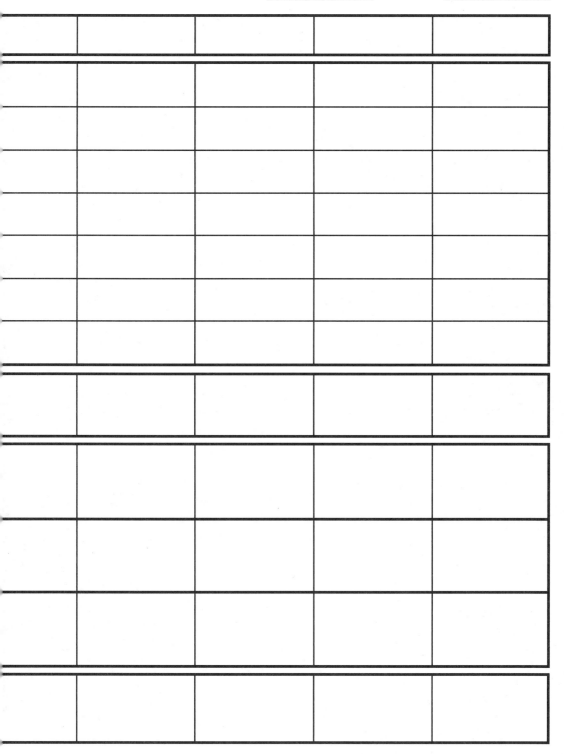

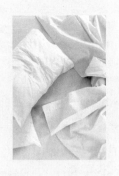

Chapter 12

Moving From Week 1 to Week 2:
Adjusting Your Bedtime

This chapter guides you forward after your first week of Sleep Therapy. I'll also show you how Julie did.

THE FIRST WEEK IS DONE

Congratulations! You made it through the first week. This is exciting. You're well on your way to good sleep. Julie found that the most difficult part of the first week was staying up later than she was used to. She had been an early-to-bed person since childhood. So this was a huge change. She loved reading but found she could not read during her long evenings because it would make her very sleepy. She tried watching some television and playing computer games but she got bored, although she did manage to do some paperwork that needed to be done.

Everyone finds her/his own thing to do to stay awake until the threshold bedtime. Some people wash dishes, some watch television, some pay bills, some play solitaire. Some tidy closets, and some even delve into art projects. One client brought in ceramic objects d'art that she had created by smashing old vases and cups and gluing the pieces in architectural designs on boards, while she was staying up until her threshold bedtime of 3 a.m.! Julie did not have so much fun, but she did see the benefits of staying up until her own threshold bedtime. She was impressed with how quickly she started to have solid sleep. Her husband noticed how rested she looked. This is not necessarily typical; not everyone looks rested after the first week. Many people have solid sleep after the first week but they look and feel tired. If you are not looking rested yet, do not despair, you soon will be!

Have a look at the following important indicators to see in what ways your sleep is starting to improve. Look at this week's sleep diary and flip back to your Baseline Sleep Diary. Compared to your Baseline Sleep Diary,

- Do you fall asleep more quickly now?

- Do you have fewer awakenings?

- Are you awake for less time during the night?

- And what about your ratings of sleep quality? Have they gone up?

Julie noticed right away that her ratings of sleep quality were consistently 8 out of 10, whereas during the initial week they were mostly 4s. She also found that she was awake for a lot less time during the night now. She had some brief awakenings but nothing compared to the hours she had been awake during the initial week. She concluded that after 1 week, her sleep was much better than it had been, although it was difficult and strange for her to stay up so late. Jot down your conclusions about your own sleep during the past week:

_____

_____

_____

_____

It's now time to move on to planning Week 2 of Sleep Therapy. In order to set your threshold bedtime for the next 7 nights, you will be using your current week's data to calculate your most recent sleep efficiency.

WHAT SLEEP EFFICIENCY DID YOU ACHIEVE?

As you did for your Baseline Sleep Diary, choose a typical night from the week just past. Mark that column of your sleep diary so you know which one it is, and follow the steps here. Turn to the chart called Calculating Your Week 1 Sleep Efficiency. Now you will be copying your Sleep Diary answers to Questions 1 to 7 for your typical night into the top part of this chart. Do the calculations for A, B, C, and then D. Voila! Here is your sleep efficiency for Week 1 of Sleep Therapy.

If at any point you realize that the night you chose is not really representative of the week, then you can try another night and see how close the sleep efficiencies are. If the nights are not consistent, then you may want to calculate all 7 sleep efficiencies and take the average for the week. It is important that you get an accurate sleep efficiency that represents the week because you will be basing your next steps on this number.

Most people find that this sleep efficiency is higher than their initial sleep efficiency. If this is true for you, yahoo! This is a sign that the techniques are working well. If your current

Calculating your Week 1 Sleep Efficiency

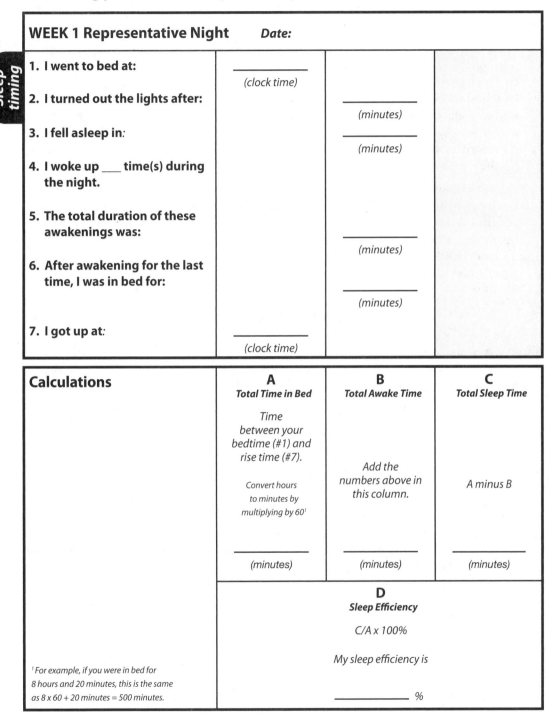

WEEK 1 Representative Night   *Date:*

Sleep timing

1. **I went to bed at:**
   _____
   (clock time)

2. **I turned out the lights after:**
   _____
   (minutes)

3. **I fell asleep in:**
   _____
   (minutes)

4. **I woke up ___ time(s) during the night.**

5. **The total duration of these awakenings was:**
   _____
   (minutes)

6. **After awakening for the last time, I was in bed for:**
   _____
   (minutes)

7. **I got up at:**
   _____
   (clock time)

Calculations

A *Total Time in Bed*	**B** *Total Awake Time*	**C** *Total Sleep Time*
Time between your bedtime (#1) and rise time (#7). *Convert hours to minutes by multiplying by 60*[1]	Add the numbers above in this column.	A minus B
_____ *(minutes)*	_____ *(minutes)*	_____ *(minutes)*

D
Sleep Efficiency

C/A x 100%

My sleep efficiency is

_____ %

[1] *For example, if you were in bed for 8 hours and 20 minutes, this is the same as 8 x 60 + 20 minutes = 500 minutes.*

sleep efficiency is *not* higher than your initial sleep efficiency, then re-do your calculations to make sure there is not a mathematical error. If you find the same results, then I suggest you do the following:

- Review how closely you have been able to follow the Six Steps to Solid Sleep. If you have not been precise with the bedtimes and rise times, or with getting out of bed when you are not sleeping, this may be reducing the benefit of the technique. Life happens, and sometimes we have family responsibilities or other activities that interfere with the timing of going to bed and getting out of bed. If this has happened, you may want to use the same threshold bedtime and rise time for another 4 days, following the instructions closely. Keep a sleep diary and re-do your sleep efficiency calculation for the 4 nights.

- Take a few moments to review the section in Chapter 1 titled Circumstances when This Book May Not Be Enough to make sure that there is not another factor that may be interfering with your sleep or your ability to benefit from this approach at this time. If something other than insomnia is causing your sleep difficulty then that "something" probably needs to be addressed first. You can always come back to Sleep Therapy after your "something" has been addressed.

ADJUSTING YOUR BEDTIME

You will now use your current sleep efficiency to determine your threshold bedtime for the upcoming week. Keep your rise time constant—the same as it was last week. Adjust your threshold bedtime according to the chart on the next page.

So, now you have your threshold bedtime for the week ahead. In the clinic, sometimes people do this calculation and get a threshold bedtime that does not seem manageable. For example, Dave had great trouble staying up until 1:00 a.m., his threshold bedtime for his first week of Sleep Therapy. His sleep efficiency for that week was 90%. According to the prescription of a new bedtime in the table on the preceding page, his new bedtime would be 15 minutes earlier (12:45 pm). However, Dave predicted this would be very difficult to do and so we discussed what would be realistic and he thought that 12:30 would be do-able. This is just to show you that you need to choose a threshold bedtime that is close to the one that is recommended but also, of course, it needs to work for you. Because I am not with you in person to look at your sleep diaries and to help you decide on the best adjustment, you will need to use your judgment to choose a new threshold bedtime that is according to the prescription, or close to it, but is also reasonable for you. After all, you will be using that bedtime all week. Usually the adjustments are 0–15 minutes per week, but sometimes they are 30 minutes. Try to avoid adjusting more than 30 minutes. This will help ensure that your sleep continues to steadily improve.

Adjusting your Threshold Bedtime

Is your sleep efficiency...	If YES,
84% or less?	Set your threshold bedtime 15 minutes *later* this week.
85% to 89%?	Keep the *same* threshold bedtime this week.
90% to 94%?	Set your threshold bedtime 15 minutes *earlier* this week.
95% or greater?	Set your threshold bedtime 30 minutes *earlier* this week.

My Week 2 threshold bedtime and rise time:

Bedtime: _____   **Rise Time:** _____

When you have decided on your new threshold bedtime for the week, record this, as well as your usual threshold rise time, in the chart Six Steps to Solid Sleep for Week 2 near the end of this chapter. Fill in your new bedtime at step 1 and your rise time at step 2. This will remind you of what you are aiming for this week.

HOW DID JULIE DO?

I will show you Julie's sleep diary and her sleep efficiency calculations as well as her decision on a new bedtime. It is often much easier to follow the steps when there is a concrete example to refer to. You may notice that near the end of the week, Julie was drifting toward an earlier bedtime. This was because she was finding it very difficult to stay up until midnight. However, she was maintaining solid sleep so the desired effect was achieved. Her homeostatic sleep process was at work. Her sleep efficiency for Saturday night was 97%. Because this was greater than 95%, she moved her threshold bedtime earlier by 30 minutes. It was midnight for Week 1, and it was set at 11:30 p.m. for Week 2.

Julie's Week 2 threshold bedtime and rise time

Bedtime: 11:30 pm   **Rise time:** 6:00 am

WEEK 1 *(Julie) Sleep Diary for the week of:* May 3

DAY of the WEEK *Which night is being reported on?*	MON.	TUES
1. I went to bed at *(clock time):*	11:45pm	11:55p
2. I turned out the lights after *(minutes):*	0	5
3. I fell asleep in *(minutes):*	5	10-1:
4. I woke up ___ time(s) during the night. *(number of awakenings):*	0	0
5. The total duration of these awakenings was *(minutes):*	0	0
6. After awakening for the last time, I was in bed for *(minutes):*	30	30
7. I got up at *(clock time):*	6:01am	6:00a
The quality of my sleep was: *1 = very poor; 10 = excellent*	8	8
Naps *Number, time and duration*	/	/
Alcohol *TIme, amount, type*	/	/
Sleep Medication *TIme, amount, type*	/	/
Notes:		hard to stay up so late

Sleep timing

Sleep quality

Bedtime: Midnight   **Rise Time:** 6:00am

NED.	THURS.	FRI.	SAT.	SUN.
:00am	12:00am	11:30pm	11:40pm	11:45pm
O	O	O	O	O
10	10	15	5	5
O	1	1	O	O
O	5 hot flashes	5 hot flashes	O	O
5	30	45	5	O
:25am	6:00am	6:00am	6:00am	6:05am
8	8	8	8	8.5
/	/	/	/	/
/	/	/	5:00pm 1 glasses of wine	/
/	/	/	/	/
Now! A od sleep				

Julie's Week 1 Sleep Efficiency

WEEK 1 Representative Night			
	Date: Sat. from Week 1		
1. I went to bed at:	<u>11:40 pm</u> *(clock time)*		
2. I turned out the lights after:		<u>0</u> *(minutes)*	
3. I feel asleep in:		<u>5</u> *(minutes)*	
4. I woke up ____ time(s) in night.			
5. The total duration of these awakenings was:		<u>0</u> *(minutes)*	
6. After awakening for the last time, I was in bed for:		<u>5</u> *(minutes)*	
7. I got up at:	<u>6:00 am</u> *(clock time)*		

Sleep timing (side tab)

Calculations	A **Total Time in Bed**	B **Total awake time**	C **Total sleep time**
	Time between your bedtime (#1) and rise time (#7). Convert hours to minutes by multiplying by 60[1]	Add the numbers above in this column	A minus B
6 hours + 20 mins = (6 × 60) + 20 = 380	<u>380</u> *(minutes)*	<u>10</u> *(minutes)*	<u>370</u> *(minutes)*
		D **Sleep Efficiency** C/A × 100% My sleep efficiency is <u>97</u> %	

[1]For example, if you were in bed for 8 hours and 20 minutes, this is the same as 8 × 60 + 20 minutes = 500 minutes.

WEEK 2

This week you will be following the Six Steps to Solid Sleep again, using your new threshold bedtime. The steps are the same as before, apart from the adjusted bedtime.

Six Steps to Solid Sleep

1. Go to bed only when sleepy and not before your threshold bedtime. _____
Fill in the threshold bedtime that you are now setting for Week 2.

2. Maintain a regular threshold rise time in the morning. _____
Fill in your threshold rise time (usually the same as before).

3. Use the bed only for sleeping. Sexual activity is the only exception. Do not watch television, listen to the radio, use electronic devices, eat, or read in bed.

4. Leave the bed if you can't fall asleep or go back to sleep within 10–15 minutes. Return when sleepy. Repeat this step as often as necessary during the night.

5. If sleepiness is overwhelming, you may take a short nap (no longer than 1 hour) in the afternoon, starting before 3 p.m.

6. Maintain a sleep diary.

Now it's time to turn to the next blank sleep diary (Week 2) and label it with the date. Then put your new threshold bedtime and rise time at the top. Having these times at the top of the sleep diary will make it easy for you to remember your mission. Keep track of your sleep for the next 7 days using this diary. Go for it!

Reminders

- Get out of bed as soon as you wake up in the morning. This applies to the situation of waking up in the morning earlier than your threshold rise time. For example, Julie woke one day at 5:30 and her threshold rise time was 6:00 a.m. She got out of bed at 5:30 a.m. and started her day. Otherwise she would have spent 30 minutes in bed awake, which would have worked against her efforts to associate her bed with sleep.

- Remember to follow the Six Steps to Solid Sleep, which include getting out of bed if you are awake for more than 10-15 minutes during the night. Return when you are sleepy.

These are probably the most common things I remind people of when they are heading into their second week of Sleep Therapy. This is refining your sleep program. Good luck this week.

WEEK 2 Sleep Diary for the week of: _____

DAY of the WEEK *Which night is being reported on?*		
1. I went to bed at *(clock time):*		
2. I turned out the lights after *(minutes):*		
3. I fell asleep in *(minutes):*		
4. I woke up ___ time(s) during the night. *(number of awakenings):*		
5. The total duration of these awakenings was *(minutes):*		
6. After awakening for the last time, I was in bed for *(minutes):*		
7. I got up at *(clock time):*		
The quality of my sleep was: *1 = very poor; 10 = excellent*		
Naps *Number, time and duration*		
Alcohol *TIme, amount, type*		
Sleep Medication *TIme, amount, type*		
Notes:		

Sleep timing (side label)
Sleep quality (side label)

Moving From Week 1 to Week 2: Adjusting Your Bedtime

Bedtime: _____ **Rise Time:** _____

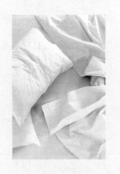

Chapter 13

Moving From Week 2 to Week 3:
Readjusting Your Bedtime

This chapter guides you forward after your second week of Sleep Therapy. Of course, I'll also let you know how Julie did.

THE SECOND WEEK IS DONE

Congratulations! You completed the second week. This is SO exciting! There will be only 1 or 2 more weeks to go of staying up late. If you didn't stay up until precisely the threshold bedtime every night, don't worry. Because of sleepiness, social events, work, children, and other demands it is very difficult to be absolutely perfect with the schedule. I find that people are often very concerned about this, but if they are close to their threshold bedtime and rise time most of the nights of the week, then they do very well. After all, you are not in a research study, you are living your life, and you don't have to be perfect.

Look over your sleep diary for the week and make some observations.

- How quickly are you falling asleep?

- How many times are you waking up?

- How long are you awake during the night?

- How are your ratings of sleep quality?

_____

_____

_____

_____

WHAT SLEEP EFFICIENCY DID YOU ACHIEVE?

As you have been doing, choose a typical night from the past week. Mark that column of your sleep diary so you know which one it is. Turn to the chart called Calculating Your Week 2 Sleep Efficiency. Now you will be copying your sleep diary answers to Questions 1 to 7 for your typical night into the top section of this chart. Do the calculations for A, B, C, and then D. Now you will have your sleep efficiency for Week 2 of Sleep Therapy.

If you are not sure if the night you chose is typical, you can always choose another one and compare the results. Pick the one that seems the most representative. Once you settle on an estimate of your current sleep efficiency, you will now set your threshold bedtime for the upcoming week. Keep your threshold rise time constant—the same as it was last week. Adjust your threshold bedtime according to the following chart.

Adjusting your Threshold Bedtime

Is your sleep efficiency	If YES,
84% or less?	Set your threshold bedtime 15 minutes *later* this week.
85% to 89%?	Keep the **same** threshold bedtime this week.
90% to 94%?	Set your threshold bedtime 15 minutes *earlier* this week.
95% or greater?	Set your threshold bedtime 30 minutes *earlier* this week.

My Week 3 threshold bedtime and rise time:

Bedtime: _____   *Rise Time:* _____

Calculating your Week 2 Sleep Efficiency

Sleep timing

WEEK 2 Representative Night	**Date:**		
1. I went to bed at:	_____ (clock time)		
2. I turned out the lights after:		_____ (minutes)	
3. I fell asleep in:		_____ (minutes)	
4. I woke up ____ time(s) during the night.			
5. The total duration of these awakenings was:		_____ (minutes)	
6. After awakening for the last time, I was in bed for:		_____ (minutes)	
7. I got up at:	_____ (clock time)		

Calculations	**A** Total Time in Bed	**B** Total Awake Time	**C** Total Sleep Time
	Time between your bedtime (#1) and rise time (#7). Convert hours to minutes by multiplying by 60[1]	Add the numbers above in this column	A minus B
	_____ (minutes)	_____ (minutes)	_____ (minutes)

	D Sleep Efficiency
[1] For example, if you were in bed for 8 hours and 20 minutes, this is the same as 8 x 60 + 20 minutes = 500 minutes.	C/Ax100% My sleep efficiency is _____ %

When you have decided on your new threshold bedtime for the week, record this, and your usual threshold rise time in the chart Six Steps to Solid Sleep for Week 3.

HOW DID JULIE DO?

Julie found that her sleep continued to improve. In Week 2 she had very few awakenings during the night and her ratings of sleep quality were mainly 7s and 8s. She found that a bedtime of 11:30 p.m. still felt very late. However, she discovered that she could use the extra time for doing some writing—a creative endeavor—that she had not found time to do for several years. That made it easier.

Julie calculated her sleep efficiency for Wednesday; it was 81%. Then she realized that she had woken up earlier that morning than most other mornings, so she chose another night as her typical night. She chose Saturday, which seemed more typical and calculated a sleep efficiency of 93%. Based on this, she advanced her bedtime (moved it earlier) by 15 minutes, to 11:15 p.m. This was just fine with her, because she had found it tough to stay up until 11:30.

Julie's Week 3 threshold bedtime and rise time:

Bedtime: 11:15pm   **Rise Time:** 6:00am

WEEK 3

Time to move on to Week 3! Just like last week, you will be following the Six Steps to Solid Sleep.

Six Steps to Solid Sleep

1. Go to bed only when sleepy and not before your threshold bedtime. _____
Fill in the threshold bedtime that you are now setting for Week 3.

2. Maintain a regular threshold rise time in the morning. _____
Fill in your threshold rise time (usually the same as before).

3. Use the bed only for sleeping. Sexual activity is the only exception. Do not watch television, listen to the radio, use electronic devices, eat, or read in bed.

4. Leave the bed if you can't fall asleep or go back to sleep within 10–15 minutes. Return when sleepy. Repeat this step as often as necessary during the night.

5. If sleepiness is overwhelming, you may take a short nap (no longer than 1 hour) in the afternoon, starting before 3 p.m.

6. Maintain a sleep diary.

You are now well acquainted with the process: Do your best to stay up until your threshold bedtime and to get up at your threshold rise time. Move to the next sleep diary form (Week 3), put in the date, and record your latest threshold bedtime and rise time at the top of the diary. Keep track of your sleep using this form for the next 7 days. Good luck.

WEEK 3 Sleep Diary for the week of: ____________

DAY of the WEEK *Which night is being reported on?*			
Sleep timing	**1. I went to bed at** *(clock time):*		
	2. I turned out the lights after *(minutes):*		
	3. I fell asleep in *(minutes):*		
	4. I woke up ___ time(s) during the night. *(number of awakenings):*		
	5. The total duration of these awakenings was *(minutes):*		
	6. After awakening for the last time, I was in bed for *(minutes):*		
	7. I got up at *(clock time):*		
Sleep quality	**The quality of my sleep was:** *1 = very poor; 10 = excellent*		
	Naps *Number, time and duration*		
	Alcohol *TIme, amount, type*		
	Sleep Medication *TIme, amount, type*		
	Notes:		

Moving From Week 2 To Week 3: Readjusting Your Bedtime

Bedtime:_____ Rise Time:_____

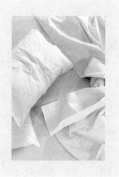

Chapter 14

After Week 3: Adjusting Your Bedtime Again. This Should Be It!

This chapter guides you forward after your third week of Sleep Therapy. Again, I'll let you know how Julie did.

THE THIRD WEEK IS DONE

Congratulations! You made it through your third week, and I bet your sleep is looking pretty good right now. Julie was finding that her sleep was good most nights. On 3 nights she slept right through without awakening and on the other 4 nights she had one brief (5-10 minute) awakening. She had one bad night—when she was awake for about 60 minutes before falling asleep and then she awakened early at 3:15 a.m.—but this was the exception. The other nights were very good.

WHAT SLEEP EFFICIENCY DID YOU ACHIEVE?

You are now at the point of making smaller adjustments to your bedtime. This is fine tuning. As you have been doing, choose a typical night from the past week, mark that column of your sleep diary. Enter your sleep diary answers for Questions 1 to 7 in the top section of the chart called Calculating Your Week 3 Sleep Efficiency. Calculate A, B, C, and then D—your sleep efficiency.

Calculating Your Week 3 Sleep Efficiency

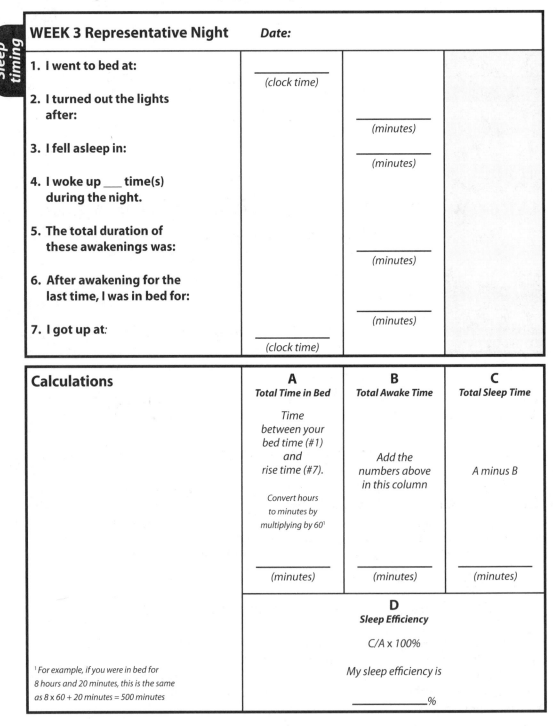

Sleep timing

WEEK 3 Representative Night   *Date:*

1. **I went to bed at:**
    _____
    (clock time)

2. **I turned out the lights after:**
    _____
    (minutes)

3. **I fell asleep in:**
    _____
    (minutes)

4. **I woke up ___ time(s) during the night.**

5. **The total duration of these awakenings was:**
    _____
    (minutes)

6. **After awakening for the last time, I was in bed for:**
    _____
    (minutes)

7. **I got up at:**
    _____
    (clock time)

Calculations	**A** *Total Time in Bed*	**B** *Total Awake Time*	**C** *Total Sleep Time*
	Time between your bed time (#1) and rise time (#7). *Convert hours to minutes by multiplying by 60[1]*	*Add the numbers above in this column*	*A minus B*
	_____ *(minutes)*	_____ *(minutes)*	_____ *(minutes)*

	D *Sleep Efficiency*
[1] *For example, if you were in bed for 8 hours and 20 minutes, this is the same as 8 x 60 + 20 minutes = 500 minutes*	*C/A x 100%* *My sleep efficiency is* _____%

Keep your threshold rise time constant and adjust your threshold bedtime according to the chart below.

Adjusting your Threshold Bedtime

Is Your Sleep Efficiency...	If YES,
84% or less?	Set your threshold bedtime 15 minutes **later** this week.
85% to 89%?	Keep the **same** threshold bedtime this week.
90% to 94%?	Set your threshold bedtime 15 minutes **earlier** this week.
95% or greater?	Set your threshold bedtime 30 minutes **earlier** this week.

My Week 4 threshold bedtime and rise time:

Bedtime: _____   Rise Time: _____

As before, write in your threshold bedtime and rise time in the chart called Six Steps to Solid Sleep (p. 93) for the upcoming week.

HOW DID JULIE DO?

Julie chose Saturday night for her calculations and got a sleep efficiency of 86%. She decided to maintain her bedtime at 11:15 and her rise time at 6:00 because her sleep was consistently good and she was not feeling sleep deprived. She calculated that she was getting about 360 minutes, or 6 hours, of sleep per night and that was enough for her to feel rested the next day.

Julie's Week 4 threshold bedtime and rise time:

Bedtime: <u>11:15pm</u>   Rise Time: <u>6:00am</u>

YOUR OVERALL PROGRESS

This is a good time to look over other aspects of your current sleep diary and compare them with your BASELINE sleep diary. Compared to your baseline week,

● Do you fall asleep more quickly now?

● Do you have fewer awakenings?

● Are you awake for less time during the night?

● And what about your ratings of sleep quality? Have they gone up?

● Are you getting more sleep than you did before?

_____

_____

_____

_____

Julie found that she was getting a bit more sleep than she had initially, and it was of much better quality. Reflecting on the changes in her sleep over the past 3 weeks, she was surprised that she only needed 6 hours of sleep per night. She had always believed that she needed more sleep than other people. Now she realized that she needed *less* sleep than many people and that it was okay to sleep for "only" 6 hours.

Julie had been tired over the past year, and she had been going to bed earlier and earlier to try and get more sleep. She had grown up with and learned to believe the rhyme: "Early to bed, early to rise makes a man healthy, wealthy and wise." However, the "early to bed" strategy had not improved her sleep. Rather, a later-to-bed strategy, based on Sleep Therapy, was the answer. Not only did her sleep improve, but her daytime fatigue lifted. Other people noticed that she looked more rested than she had for some time. Her husband thought she was a changed person. She was not entirely sure if this was a compliment or not, but she guessed it probably was!

MOVING ON FROM HERE

By now, you have the know-how to continue to adjust your bedtime week by week if needed. You may need to make small adjustments of your threshold bedtime until your sleep, on almost all nights of the week, is of high quality and long enough so that you are refreshed and not sleepy the next day. Once this is reached, you will have discovered your own optimal sleep duration for this point in your life. Once again, congratulations.

Julie continued to have a regular bedtime of about 11:15 p.m., and got up at 6:00 a.m.—this worked for her and she was satisfied with her sleep. Even though she continued to have some awakenings (e.g., for the bathroom or due to hot flashes), she was able to go back to sleep quickly. She told me: "I don't worry anymore about falling asleep. I have trust in falling asleep." Overall, she was more relaxed about her sleep.

At this point Julie was wondering how to maintain her good sleep; she was a bit afraid that it would not last. Naturally, you may be wondering the same thing. It is important to know that you will be able to keep your good sleep going. You have learned the most important principles and steps that can always be applied to improve your sleep. It is helpful to set up a specific maintenance plan for yourself. Chapter 17 will guide you through this, allowing you to feel confident in your ability to maintain your good sleep.

WEEK 4 AND BEYOND

Here are your Six Steps to Solid Sleep. Insert your threshold bedtime and rise time for Week 4. You are probably close to a bedtime that is best for you at this point in your life.

Six Steps to Solid Sleep

1. Go to bed only when sleepy and not before your threshold bedtime._____
Fill in the threshold bedtime that you are now setting for the upcoming week.

2. Maintain a regular threshold rise time in the morning. _____
Fill in your threshold rise time (usually the same as before).

3. Use the bed only for sleeping. Sexual activity is the only exception. Do not watch television, listen to the radio, use electronic devices, eat, or read in bed.

4. Leave the bed if you can't fall asleep or go back to sleep within 10–15 minutes. Return when sleepy. Repeat this step as often as necessary during the night.

5. If sleepiness is overwhelming, you may take a short nap (no longer than 1 hour) in the afternoon, starting before 3 p.m.

6. Maintain a sleep diary.

You will find a blank sleep diary for Week 4 at the end of the chapter. After that, if you continue to monitor your sleep, feel free to copy a blank Sleep Diary from Appendix B. Also in Appendix B you will find blank charts for calculating your sleep efficiency. These charts and your know-how will serve you well if your insomnia ever returns.

WEEK 4 Sleep Diary for the week of: _____

DAY of the WEEK *Which night is being reported on?*		
Sleep timing		
1. I went to bed at *(clock time):*		
2. I turned out the lights after *(minutes):*		
3. I fell asleep in *(minutes):*		
4. I woke up ___ time(s) during the night. *(number of awakenings):*		
5. The total duration of these awakenings was *(minutes):*		
6. After awakening for the last time, I was in bed for *(minutes):*		
7. I got up at *(clock time):*		
Sleep quality — **The quality of my sleep was:** *1 = very poor; 10 = excellent*		
Naps *Number, time and duration*		
Alcohol *Time, amount, type*		
Sleep Medication *Time, amount, type*		
Notes:		

After Week 3: Adjusting Your Bedtime Again. This Should Be It!

Bedtime: _____ **Rise Time:** _____

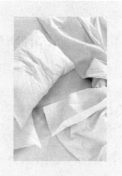

Chapter 15

Do You Still Have Insomnia?

After Week 4 of Sleep Therapy, or when you are fairly satisfied with your threshold bedtime and you know the routine—the Six Steps to Solid Sleep—inside out, I suggest that you check to see if you are now free from insomnia. You can do this by looking at the same things in your current sleep diary that you did in Chapter 7, before you started Sleep Therapy.

INITIAL INSOMNIA

Take your eye across your current sleep diary at Question 3 and see how long it took you to fall asleep each night. Did it often (on 3 nights or more) take you longer than 30 minutes to fall asleep? If so, you are experiencing "initial insomnia" and you can circle "initial insomnia" in the right-hand column of the chart with the question "What Type of Insomnia Do I have Now?" on the next page.

MULTIPLE AWAKENINGS

Cast your eye across your current sleep diary at Question 4. Look at the number of awakenings you had each night. Did you often (on 3 nights or more) have more than 3 awakenings per night? If so, you can describe yourself as having "multiple awakenings." If you answered yes, then circle "multiple awakenings" in the right-hand column of the chart with the question "What Type of Insomnia Do I Have Now?" on the next page.

MIDDLE INSOMNIA

Look at how long you were awake each night, which is at Question 5. Is this number often (3 nights or more) greater than 30 minutes? If so, you are experiencing "middle insomnia." If this applies to you, then circle "middle insomnia" in the right-hand column of the chart with the question "What Type of Insomnia Do I Have Now?" on the next page.

TERMINAL (END-OF-NIGHT) INSOMNIA

Look over the times that you were awake in bed in the morning at Question 6. Was this often (3 nights or more) 30 minutes or longer? If so, was this because you woke up earlier than you had wanted? Do not count any mornings that you purposely lay in bed awake rather than getting up. Just count the mornings you woke up too early by more than 30 minutes. If you are waking up more than 30 minutes too early on at least 3 mornings, then you have "terminal" or "end-of-night" insomnia, so circle "terminal insomnia" in the right-hand column of the chart with the question "What Type of Insomnia Do I Have Now?" on the next page.

YOUR SLEEP QUALITY

On your current sleep diary, look at your sleep quality ratings across the days of the week. Take your most common rating. If, in Chapter 7, rather than having a "most common rating," you calculated an average rating, then calculate your new average sleep quality rating now. Record your most common rating (or the average) in the chart on the next page where it says "The Quality of My Sleep Now."

YOUR PROGRESS

Take a long and careful look at this chart, and the same one in Chapter 7, p. 39. In comparing your answers to the same questions at baseline, what do you conclude? You probably deserve a giant pat on the back about now.

After Sleep Therapy:

What type of Insomnia do I have now?	Circle all that apply
Long time to get to sleep (more than 30 minutes)	**Initial Insomnia**
Many awakenings (more than 3)	**Multiple Awakenings**
Long time awake during the night (more than 30 minutes)	**Middle Insomnia**
Waking up too early (more than 30 minutes)	**Terminal Insomnia**
The quality of my sleep now	Most common rating now: _____

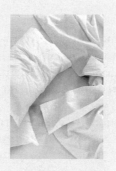

Chapter 16

What to Do With Your Mind

"A ruffled mind makes a restless pillow."

Charlotte Brontë

As I write this, it is August and I am on vacation. I am sitting on a porch that looks out on a bay of the Northumberland Strait in Nova Scotia. In front of me are sand dunes, packed with tall bright green grasses that are swaying in the breeze. Beyond the sand dunes is a great expanse of water, blue, and gray. It is early morning and the tide is going out, exposing fawn-colored, rippled sand. The sky is mostly clear, but there are some small fluffy clouds. The air is soft and warm; the breeze feels gentle. Over to the right, along the beach, where the sea meets the sand, I see a great blue heron—a tall, thin bird with stick-like legs and long beak, waiting to see something appetizing in the water. To my left, about 200 meters in the distance, is a narrow spit of sand, which is becoming more and more exposed as the tide recedes. On this spit are six seals, sunning themselves, and periodically slipping into the water. I notice a hummingbird when it buzzes near me, flitting through the fragrant wild rose bushes next to the porch. You may have a feel of the place by now. Do you?

Your ability to have a feel of this place demonstrates that you can take your mind to places that are different from where your mind was before. You can lead your mind to places of your choosing. And just by noticing this foray, by responding to my question "Do you?" you are stepping back from your normal thoughts and assuming an "observer's mind," an ability to be aware of what your mind is doing—where it is, what types of thoughts and images are there. These two abilities—taking your mind to places that you choose, and having an observer's mind—are very useful skills to develop.

Developing these skills allows room for the "velvet hammer" of sleep to descend. Velvet hammer is a term used by a man who described to me how sleep had returned to him after a long bout of insomnia. He said a wee angel had gently knocked him on the head with a velvet hammer and this had restored his sleep. I like this image because it reflects the nature of sleep: It comes of its own accord, and not when we are searching for it. All we can do is to make the conditions conducive to sleep arriving and then leave the rest to our natural sleep processes. Overactive mental activity can be a big barrier to the velvet hammer, but it is one that is malleable.

THE RACING MIND

I often hear "My mind won't shut off." "I wish I could switch off my brain." Many people with insomnia describe having racing thoughts at night. These thoughts are sometimes centered on topics of stress, trying to solve problems. Other times the thoughts seem to be all over the place, not focused on specific issues; the mind flits from topic to topic. Naturally, an active mind interferes with sleep arriving; it prevents the velvet hammer from descending. What to do with this active mind?

There are several helpful strategies for calming active thoughts. To begin with, it is helpful to take an observer's stance, and notice where exactly your mind is going. Tonight, observe where your mind is when you are not sleeping. You may want to jot down your observations on a note pad next to the bed. The next day, look at your list.

Thoughts or Worries About the Effects of Not Sleeping

Is your mind going to thoughts about not sleeping? Are there worries about what will happen if you don't sleep? If this is the case, you can rest assured that with Sleep Therapy, which is CBT-I, you are using the best treatment that exists for insomnia, and that is all you need to do right now. You can also reassure yourself that the effects of not sleeping, or hardly sleeping, for one night are more subtle than you might think. Refer back to Chapter 3 for specific information that can ground your thoughts in reality. It is common for our fears and worries to expand and to become all-consuming in the middle of the night. In the light of day, you can adjust and balance this thinking. Then, when the same worries come up at night, you can remind yourself of the less-distressing facts and invite in your more realistic thoughts on the topic.

Let's look at an example. When Julie was working at her administrative job, she was acutely aware of the effects of not sleeping on her ability to do her job well. She needed to be on top of things, and to think clearly in order to make good decisions and interact with people effectively. At night she worried: "If I don't sleep tonight, I won't be able to function tomorrow. I will perform poorly and it will be terrible." After Julie evaluated this prediction, and after she learned more about the actual effects on performance of not sleeping, she came up with an alternate belief. Her new belief was: "I may not feel at the top of my game if I don't sleep, but I can still function at work and get through the day okay." This new thought was accompanied by much less apprehension and was actually a rather boring thought. This realistic thought was less of a barrier to the velvet hammer.

I often find that once people follow the Six Steps to Solid Sleep—the methods outlined in the previous chapters—they often do not need to deal anymore with worrisome thoughts about sleep. This is perhaps because they are absorbed in carrying out the techniques, or perhaps they are too sleepy to worry, or they have less time in bed to think about not sleeping, or they have experienced the good sleep that comes from using Sleep Therapy. Whatever the particular reason, using the Sleep Therapy techniques often relieves people of worries about not sleeping. If you are just starting to use the Six Steps and you are still having some sleep-related worries, try reassuring yourself that: a) you are using the most effective techniques to sleep well already, and you need only to follow the instructions and leave the rest to your internal sleep processes; and b) all of us, including you, can only experience life one moment at a time, and so we have no ability right now to influence all those previous nights of poor sleep or any anticipated future nights of poor sleep. So you can drop worries about those past and future nights. You have only this night that you can influence. We know that nothing horrible happens after one night of complete sleep loss (see Chapter 3) so there is no need for alarm, even if you are up all night.

Trying to Sleep

Sometimes we try too hard to sleep. If you have ever told someone, "I was lying there, trying to sleep" or something similar, this implies that you are taking too much responsibility for controlling sleep. It is like trying to find happiness. Once we look too hard for it, it eludes us. It cannot be forced. Rather, it arrives when we are open to it, but not searching for it. So, you may be wondering what can I do then, if I don't *try* to sleep? The answer is: Just make the conditions good enough for your sleep processes to operate, using the sleep scheduling procedures of Sleep Therapy, and then let them do their thing. As you recall, if you haven't slept within about 10–15 minutes, get out of bed and do something. Return when you feel the physical signs of sleepiness. No need to think about it.

If you find that despite all this, you still feel you need to control your sleep, then this performance pressure may be the very thing that is preventing the velvet hammer of sleep from descending. For some people, this anxiety is lifted when they actually reverse what they are trying to do. Rather than trying to sleep, they *try to stay awake*. This is called "paradoxical intention." If you feel you "must" sleep or "have to get to sleep" or you are "trying" hard to sleep, then give paradoxical intention a try, and see how long you can stay awake. Just by releasing the pressure on yourself to sleep, your internal sleep processes will be better able to do what they are designed to do—bring on sleep.

Worries About Things Going on in Your Life

Is your mind going to worries about things that are happening in your life right now? It is very common to have worries about work, school, relationships, family, or health issues. If this is true for you, then write these issues down on paper during the daytime. Then consider which are productive worries and which are nonproductive. For example, if I am stressed about a deadline for a paper, this is a productive worry because I can start brain-storming to develop a plan for meeting the deadline or extending it.

That is, I can probably use problem-solving techniques to resolve it. Whereas, if I am worried about what I said in a conversation and wish I had expressed myself more clearly, or if I have a large mortgage to pay down and know that it will take several years and there are vague uncertainties about my job prospects in 5 years, these are examples of nonproductive worries. It doesn't matter how much time I put my mind on them, I cannot resolve them right now. As you might imagine, nonproductive worry takes energy and brain power but goes nowhere. It also adds to our frustration as we go round and round without a solution. These are the worries that you can learn to release and set free.

For productive worries

A technique that many people find helpful is called "Worry Time." I like to call it "Clear-Your-Head Time" because it can also be used for recurring thoughts, plans, or issues that you might not call "worries" exactly. Clear-Your-Head Time involves sitting down in the evening with a notebook, a sheet of paper, or a set of blank index cards, and writing down all the things that come to mind, or are likely to come to mind, later that night in bed. You do this early in the evening, at least 2 hours prior to bedtime. After you have gotten all those issues out of your head and on paper (point form is good enough), then you come up with a solution, at least a temporary one, for each issue. You need to come up with something that will put that issue to rest for the night. For most issues, you will not be solving the whole thing during your Clear-Your-Head Time, you will just be deciding on what you do with that issue for the night. Solutions are things like: "I will phone Tim about that tomorrow at lunchtime." Or "I can't do anything more about that tonight so I will think about it some more tomorrow evening from 7:00–7:30." This is a way of putting your issues to bed early so that they don't pop up to disturb your sleep. If they *do* pop into your mind later while you are in bed, you can remind yourself that you have dealt with the issue(s) for the night and there is nothing left to work on now. All is well.

Sometimes, things we have not anticipated—other issues—come into our heads while we are in bed. This is when I grab a piece of paper next to the bed and write down a word or two that summarizes the unanticipated issue and tell myself that I will deal with it tomorrow during my Clear-Your-Head Time. You may want to keep a blank sheet of paper or card with a pen next to your bed for this purpose.

For nonproductive worries or miscellaneous thoughts

Nonproductive thoughts and worries are things that can be released and let go of at night. More easily said than done, I know. I find that the best way to release these thoughts is to use visual imagery. By this I mean you will be using your ability to imagine things in your mind's eye, just as you were able to see the scene at the Nova Scotia shore even though you weren't there at the time. I will give you some examples of useful methods that you can try.

For thoughts that go round and round in your head and are getting you nowhere, you can imagine each thought, or group of thoughts, being engulfed by a bubble which then floats upward into the sky. When I was having trouble letting go of certain patterns of thought that were interfering with my sleep a few years ago, I tried the bubble imagery. However, my bubble was too fragile and I saw it bursting and not doing the job of carrying away my thoughts. So I then imagined a more resilient bubble—more like a rubber ball—enclosing my thoughts. I envisioned myself whacking this ball with a baseball bat into outer space. That was fine for a few seconds. But then my ball-balloon went right around Earth and returned from behind me! I was annoyed, but also amused. I then batted it again. This time it went around Earth, passed by me, and soared over the ocean. I then saw it fall and break into pieces as it hit the water. The pieces descended into the depths, becoming finer and finer as they sank toward the bottom of the sea. Along the way, the biodegradable pieces were eaten by fish until there was nothing left. Then, finally, I felt satisfied that I had let go of those thoughts! So you see that you can use your imagination to let go of even very stubborn thoughts. It's like this quote from Mark Twain: "Drag your thoughts away from your troubles ... by the ears, by the heels, or any other way you can manage."

Some people find it very helpful to "shelve" their thoughts for the night. They figuratively put them on the top shelf of a cupboard, often in a box. You can make it a shoe box, a square box, a hat box, or whatever size and shape of box you wish. The box can be whatever colour or pattern that you imagine. The main thing is that you put away your thoughts in this safe place, where they can always be retrieved at another time (or not). You can have some fun with the details of this shelving process. Your imagination is the limit.

What to Do With Your Mind After You Have Let the Issues Go?

You may now be wondering, "What do I do now that I have let go of the issues that were on my mind?" I suggest you take your mind into your sock drawer and see if you can see how your socks are arranged in there. Really! What do your socks look like? How do they sit in the drawer? Or you might want to imagine waves rolling in, and looking at each wave as it moves toward the shore. You could imagine looking at clouds in the sky and seeing shapes in them. Basically, occupying your mind with images is a way to step off the over-active-thinking train. You want images that are pleasant and somewhat boring. For some reason, counting sheep as they jump over a fence does not seem to help many people. However, you could imagine a flock of sheep standing in a field, and one after another, lying down to sleep. Did you know that sheep first drop down on their "elbows" and then lower their behinds?

Sleep researchers have found that, as we drift off to sleep, we have what's called "hypnagogic mentation," which is most often fleeting visual images. These images are moving and may include shape patterns of things we have recently been watching. I have a hunch—this has not yet been scientifically tested—that if your mind is already in a visual mode, rather than a problem-solving, thinking mode, your brain is in a state more conducive to sleep arriving. So, when I have trouble sleeping, I try to go to visual images when I'm in bed, and do my thinking when I'm out of bed.

DEVELOPING AN OBSERVER'S MIND

Another approach to get out of problem-solving mode, or overactive-thinking mode, is by training your mind with meditation. There are many types of meditation and you can choose the type that suits you best. In meditation, we learn how to focus the mind on one thing, letting other thoughts and mental events float away. I will introduce you to "mindfulness" meditation. I find it is an antidote to today's fast-paced, multi-tasking world. *Mindfulness is about being aware in the present moment and without judgment.* I will describe formal practice and informal practice. If you are new to meditation, then I suggest you start by doing formal practice during the daytime, sitting up. After you are comfortable with the methods, then you might do some informal mindfulness practice when you are awake in bed at night. (However, remember that you should never be awake in bed for longer than about 15 minutes.)

Formal Mindfulness Practice

Formal mindfulness practice involves setting aside some time each day to focus the mind. Start by sitting comfortably, in a dignified posture, and focusing on the physical sensations of your breath. Without altering your breathing, simply observe it. You could choose to be aware of your chest or abdomen rising and falling, you could be aware of the sound of your breath, notice the sensation of the air as it enters the nostrils, or the air as it leave the nostrils or the mouth. You might pay attention to the rate or depth of your breathing, or the period between each breath. Choose one of the many aspects of your breathing and focus your attention there. Your breath is always with you so it is an ideal focus that can be used anywhere, any time. Throughout history, people have used the breath to focus the mind. If you are really focusing, you may notice that one breath is different from the next, and you may notice aspects of your breath that you have never noticed before. There is no need to adjust your breathing to make it deeper or slower; simply observe what you find.

Some people find that they do not like focusing on the breath. For people in the clinic who are uncomfortable with this, I usually suggest that they notice the physical sensations of one hand clasped in the other, on their lap. So as you are sitting, you would notice the touch of one hand on the other, the points of contact, the warmth, the heaviness, and so on.

An important part of any meditation is noticing thoughts or sounds or pains that distract us from the focus. It is completely normal to be distracted. Our minds are meant to wander. So, the idea is to accept these wanderings, and when you notice them, gently guide your mind back to the focus. It is important to do so kindly, without judgment. At first, you may have to do this hundreds of times during a formal practice. That's entirely fine. It's good to notice these distractions—that is part of the awareness. You are developing your observer's mind. You could start with 5 minutes of formal practice and work up to 20 minutes per day. You can guide yourself using the exercise here, or play a mindfulness recording so that someone's voice guides you through. Mindfulness meditation recordings are available commercially. Over time and with experience, you will probably find that you do not need printed or recorded instructions anymore; you will be guiding yourself in formal practice.

A starter exercise in Mindfulness Meditation Practice

- Set aside 5 minutes when you won't be interrupted.
- Sit in a chair, with your feet grounded on the floor.
- Assume a dignified posture.
- Close your eyes and become aware of your breath.
- To cue your awareness of your breath, you could start with a sigh or a release of air, and then notice the re-filling of your lungs. Notice how the belly rises as air comes in.
- Follow each subsequent breath and pay attention to your belly rising and falling. You may start to become aware of your nostrils and how the air feels as it enters your nose and how it feels when it is released.
- As you breathe, let yourself notice whatever there is to be noticed about each breath.
- Silently count each breath, up to 10.
- Then start again at 1 and count in rounds of 10. If you lose track, start again at 1.
- Each and every time your mind is distracted from observation of the breath, gently guide your mind back to your breath.
- After 5 rounds of 10 breaths, allow your eyes to open. Notice how you feel.

Repeat each day for a week. The next week, increase your time to 10 minutes. Continue to increase the duration of your practice by 5 minutes per week, until you reach 20 minutes per day.

Informal Mindfulness Practice

Whereas formal mindfulness is a disciplined practice of setting aside a time each day to focus the mind on one thing, informal mindfulness is being aware, in our day-to-day existence, of our experience—whether it be physical sensations, our five senses, our thoughts, or our feelings. As with formal mindfulness, we do so without judgment. This sounds very big and all-encompassing, but it starts simply. It begins by just taking a minute now, whatever you happen to be doing, to be aware of how your body is, what is going through your mind, what sounds you hear, what your eyes see. Be totally immersed in the moment. Informal practice is incorporated into your everyday activities—you do whatever you are doing mindfully, rather than automatically. For instance, you might brush your teeth mindfully, wash dishes mindfully, put out the recycling and garbage mindfully, or interact with your pet mindfully. I suggest 1 minute because at first it is difficult to be totally mindful for even that length of time. As you get more practice, you will have more mindful minutes during the day. Being mindful allows us to be present now, rather than being caught up in problem-solving mode, planning mode, re-play mode, or whatever other track our minds tend to go on. It allows us to experience life from moment to moment rather than being elsewhere in our thoughts.

You can use informal mindfulness practice if you are awake in bed at night. Lying in bed, you could become aware of your breath, observing the same aspects that you observe during your formal practice during the day. If you are someone who does not like to focus on your breath, you might choose to notice other physical sensations like the points of contact between the bed and your skin, how each of those points feels physically—noticing things like warmth, softness/hardness, flatness—or notice how your legs and feet contact each other. As before, do not be disturbed by intruding thoughts, just notice them and let them go, like clouds in the sky, let them float by. And remember, get out of bed and do something if you are awake for more than 10–15 minutes.

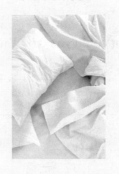

Chapter 17

Maintaining Your Progress

(And Maybe Even Improving More!)

Often people who are starting to improve their sleep worry that their progress is only temporary and that poor sleep will return. This was going through Julie's mind—she was feeling satisfied with her sleep but there was a little something telling her that this would not last. If you've had insomnia for several years, you may be especially prone to this fear of relapse. Now is the ideal time to look at maintenance strategies. Maintenance starts with reminding yourself that you have acquired new knowledge about your sleep and mastered the strategies that improve it. This is very important to remember; it means that you will never be back at "square one."

Now, let's take some very practical steps to anticipate what could happen. What is your fear? Is it that you will have a bad night? A totally sleepless night? A string of bad nights? Write down exactly what you think might happen:

_____

_____

_____

_____

Based on what you now know, what could you do if this did happen?

1. _____

2. _____

3. _____

4. _____

If you wish to get your sleep back on track, it is just a matter of recalling the Sleep Therapy steps that have already worked for you. Then, put them into action. When I ask people in my Sleep Therapy groups what they would do if they started to have some bad nights, they generally fill the whiteboard with ideas like this:

- Stay up late, past my normal bedtime.

- Get up at the same time each day.

- Keep a sleep diary.

- Use visual imagery.

- Get out of bed when I'm not sleeping.

- Don't go to bed unless I'm sleepy.

- Do clear-my-head time.

- Reassure myself that one bad night does not forecast a string of bad nights.

- Know that I will function tomorrow even if I don't have a good sleep tonight.

Sometimes we actually choose to return to old habits, like reading in bed. This is just fine; it is, of course, your choice. This happened for a short time to Julie. As you know, she was sleeping well by staying up until 11:15 p.m. This was a much later bedtime than she had been accustomed to. One day in December she told me she had "fallen off the wagon." By this she meant she had started to go to bed much earlier again because it was dark and cold outside, and she wanted to read in bed. She also felt comforted by going to bed earlier. With this resumption of early bedtimes, Julie was falling asleep fine but she was having some long awakenings during the night. At this point she decided to keep doing what she was doing for a few weeks even though she knew what to do to make her sleep continuous. She knew she just had to read in her living room rather than in bed, and to stay up later.

This is a nice example because it shows that if you have the know-how you can apply it any time you choose. I want to point out that Julie felt somewhat sheepish about "falling off the wagon," and this is a common feeling in this circumstance. I encouraged her to let go of this self-judgment. Indeed, you should do what you choose. Feeling guilty or being self-critical when you have poor sleep will serve no purpose other than to make your mind more troubled. So, have some kindness for yourself if poor sleep returns. Simply follow the Six Steps to Solid Sleep, shown on the next page, when you are ready, and your sleep will be back on track in no time!

Note that you do not have to go back to the very beginning. Use a threshold bedtime that is based on your threshold bedtime from Chapter 14: Make it 60 minutes later than that for 4-7 days. After 4-7 days, adjust your bedtime according to what your sleep diary tells you. For example, if your sleep efficiency is very high, you would advance your bedtime. You will soon get back to solid sleep. Your goal is to get back to a point where you are having solid sleep that is long enough for you to feel rested, and not sleepy, during the daytime.

In our clinic, people tend to keep sleeping well long after they complete our Sleep Therapy program. It is not uncommon for me to receive notes or cards from clients, months after the program, saying that they are still sleeping well. Also, from research we know that after people learn cognitive behavioral therapy for insomnia (CBT-I), the techniques on which Sleep Therapy is based, they continue to benefit from them. For example, Dr. Charles Morin found, in a study with people aged 55 and over, that those who did CBT-I maintained their progress very well *2 years* after they learned the techniques.

Once you know the strategies for improving sleep you can use them as needed. If you are curious about whether you can go back to some of your favorite habits like reading in bed, or sleeping in on the week-ends, and still maintain your good sleep, you can always find out. Be a scientist. Try re-introducing one behavior at a time for a week, keep sleep diaries, and see what effect it has, if any, on your sleep. You are becoming more and more tuned into your own particular sleep–wake system. You are the expert on knowing what works best to maintain your good sleep.

Six Steps to Solid Sleep

1. Go to bed only when sleepy and not before your threshold bedtime._____
Recall what your threshold bedtime was in Chapter 14 (page 93) and now make it later,
for example, by 60 minutes.

2. Maintain a regular threshold rise time in the morning. _____
Fill in the threshold rise time that you had in Chapter 14 (page 93).

3. Use the bed only for sleeping. Sexual activity is the only exception. Do not watch television, listen to the radio, use electronic devices, eat, or read in bed.

4. Leave the bed if you can't fall asleep or go back to sleep within 10–15 minutes. Return when sleepy. Repeat this step as often as necessary during the night.

5. If sleepiness is overwhelming, you may take a short nap (no longer than 1 hour) in the afternoon, starting before 3 p.m.

6. Maintain a sleep diary.

Sleep Diary for the Week of: _____

DAY of the WEEK *Which night is being reported on?*		

Sleep timing

1. I went to bed at *(clock time):*		
2. I turned out the lights after *(minutes):*		
3. I fell asleep in *(minutes):*		
4. I woke up ___ time(s) during the night. *(number of awakenings):*		
5. The total duration of these **awakenings was** *(minutes):*		
6. After awakening for the last time, **I was in bed for** *(minutes):*		
7. I got up at *(clock time):*		

Sleep quality

The quality of my sleep was: *1 = very poor; 10 = excellent*		

Naps *Number, time and duration*		
Alcohol *TIme, amount, type*		
Sleep Medication *TIme, amount, type*		
Notes:		

Bedtime: _____ Rise Time: _____

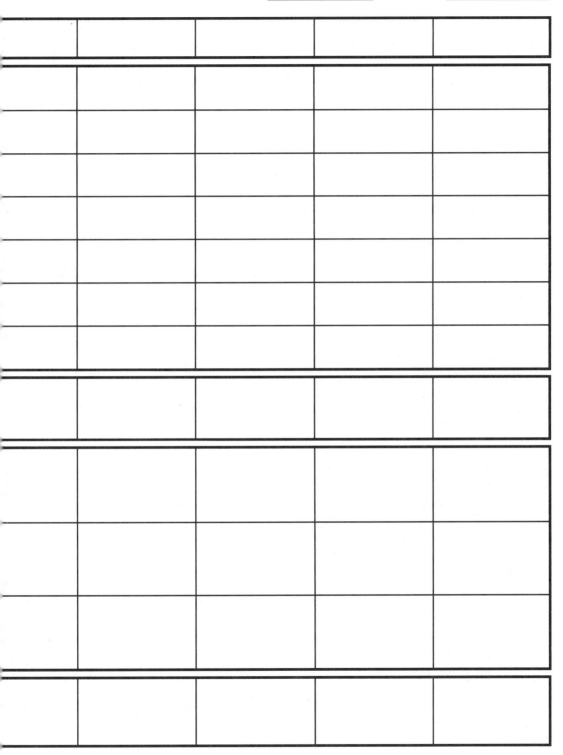

Sleep in Special Circumstances—More Hope

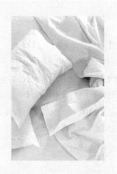

Chapter 18

You're a Woman. You Have
Special Sleep Needs

You guessed it—women are more likely than men to have insomnia. At least, they report it more often on surveys. About 11% of women have persistent insomnia that is severe enough that it interferes with their functioning, and many others are simply dissatisfied with their sleep. Some estimates are as high as 61% for the percent of women who have some kind of sleep problem. Why are the rates high in women? Well, perhaps women have greater awareness of their sleep and well-being, and perhaps they are more likely than men to acknowledge and report physical and mental distress. Biological factors may also come into play: pregnancy and menopause are times when sleep is apt to be especially disturbed. In addition, although many men are active in family caregiving, women tend to be more involved in nighttime care of babies, children, and older relatives. This nighttime vigilance for the needs of young ones and/or elders can contribute to sleeplessness, even after the children have grown up and the nighttime caregiving ends. Also, many women are pulled in several directions by demands of work, home, and family; this sets the stage for nighttime worries and problem-solving mental activity that can prevent sleep from arriving.

HOW DOES INSOMNIA START?

A family history of insomnia increases the likelihood of developing insomnia, especially if your mother had sleep difficulty. The extent to which this reflects genetic predisposition and/or the environment in which you grew up is unclear; probably it is a combination of both nature and nurture. If you, like your mother, are prone to "hyperarousal"—over-stimulation of mind and body—then you are more likely to develop insomnia. While you were growing up, if your mother did not sleep well, you may have picked up some sleep-hindering habits yourself, such as going to bed too early, having variable bedtimes and rise times, or worrying about not sleeping. Whatever the mechanism behind the influence of family history on your sleep, you are not locked into insomnia just because it runs in your family. There are many situations where the family is insomnia-prone but the person isn't, and vice versa. Also, if you do have insomnia you can certainly learn to sleep well, by using cognitive behavioral therapy for insomnia (CBT-I), the basis of Sleep Therapy, regardless of your family history.

By adolescence, about 5%–10% of girls have insomnia. A study of adolescents, age 13–16 years, in Detroit, Michigan, found that before the onset of menses, girls and boys had similar rates of insomnia. It was after girls started menstruating that their rates of insomnia climbed steeply, surpassing that of boys. Girls ended up being 2.5 times more likely to have insomnia than boys. Whether this increase in insomnia rate is linked to hormonal changes that occur at puberty in girls or to social developmental changes (e.g., young teen girls being more excited about social relationships) is unknown. This is an area we need to understand more, especially because there are signs that adolescent insomnia is not just a fleeting period of poor sleep; it tends to linger.

WHAT HAPPENS DURING YOUR MENSTRUAL CYCLE?

Some girls and women experience worse sleep in the 3–4 days before their menstrual period than at other times in their cycle. This is especially likely if you have premenstrual symptoms like depressed mood, irritability, appetite changes, and feeling tense or on edge. In most women, the sleep changes are quite subtle and may even go unnoticed. However, when periods involve pain and cramping, sleep is more obviously affected. Women with painful periods are more likely than other women to experience poor sleep, unpleasant dreams around their period, and greater sleepiness in the 2 weeks before their period.

> For painful periods, nonsteroidal anti-inflammatory medications (e.g., ibuprofen, naproxen sodium) can be helpful for both relieving the pain and improving your sleep quality.

What about sleep when you take oral contraceptives? The effects have rarely been studied, but the few bits of research show negligible differences between sleep with oral contraceptives compared to sleep without oral contraceptives.

WHAT HAPPENS WHEN YOU ARE PREGNANT?

Changes in a woman's sleep are evident within 11–12 weeks of pregnancy. This is not surprising given that the first trimester—the first 3 months of pregnancy—may bring nausea and vomiting (formerly called "morning sickness"), back pain, and a need to urinate more frequently. Women often feel fatigued and sleepy during the daytime, a phenomenon that continues throughout pregnancy. The sleepiness is probably related to the high levels of the hormone progesterone, which, in addition to protecting the lining of the uterus for the fetus, promotes sleep. Consistent with women's reports of poorer sleep quality, sleep laboratory measures show a reduction in deep sleep and an increase in number of awakenings during the first trimester.

In the second trimester—the middle 3 months of pregnancy—there is usually some relief from the nausea. Other physical pressures develop including abdominal discomfort, lower back pain, movements of the baby, pressure on the bladder, heartburn, cramps or tingling in the legs, and shortness of breath. As you can imagine, these lead to further sleep disruption and awakenings. Researchers are divided about whether deep sleep increases, decreases, or stays about the same as the pregnancy progresses. It would be nice to think that it increases, and provides super-restful sleep for the mother-to-be but this may be wishful thinking. What *is* clear is that there are more frequent awakenings as the pregnancy advances. By the third trimester—the last 3 months of pregnancy—almost all women wake up at night because of physical discomfort or a need to urinate.

> In late pregnancy, the most comfortable sleeping position may be on your side with a pillow between your knees. Try different pillow arrangements to see what is most for comfortable for you. If you are sleepy during the day and circumstances allow it, lie down for a nap.

Women are often aware of dreams during their pregnancy. It is not uncommon to have dreams about the baby; one study found that 35%–40% of pregnant women reported having such dreams. Nightmares may also occur and sometimes these disturbing dreams involve the baby being in some kind of danger. Naturally, these dreams can be alarming for the mother-to-be. They no doubt reflect normal maternal concerns about the child's safety. It may be reassuring to know that dreams do not predict the future but they may play a useful role in pregnancy. Dr. Rosalind Cartwright, one of the world's preeminent dream researchers, believes that dreams help us to regulate our emotions, and that anxious pregnancy dreams may allow the woman to rehearse responses to possible difficulties and to process the natural anxiety around labor and delivery. It is very common to have some anxiety and fear about the childbirth process. A survey from British Columbia found that 79% of women who were close to their due date (35–39 weeks pregnancy) had moderate to high levels of childbirth fear. Those women who were most fearful had more stress in their lives and had fewer people around to help. They were also likely to be fatigued and to get less sleep. Therefore, this very common type of fear during the late stages of pregnancy can sometimes lead to further sleep difficulty.

As if this "news" about sleep in pregnancy were not bad enough, pregnancy also increases the risk of developing some other sleep disorders. "Restless legs syndrome" involves leg sensations like crawling, tingling, numbness, or pain, with a feeling that you have to move your legs. These sensations are most likely to happen when you are resting or lying in bed in the evening. They usually go away with movement such as walking or stretching. At least one-quarter of pregnant women experience restless legs. No one knows for sure why pregnancy can bring on restless legs, but possibilities are the influence of reproductive hormones or low iron levels on the neurotransmitter (chemical messenger between nerve cells) dopamine, which is involved in movement control. When leg restlessness occurs, it usually starts in the third or fourth month of pregnancy and increases to a maximum in the eighth month. Interestingly, restless legs syndrome subsides in the ninth month and usually stops around the time of delivery. If you are someone who had restless legs prior to pregnancy, you can expect this problem to worsen during pregnancy and then return to pre-existing levels after the baby's birth. So how does restless legs syndrome affect sleep? Frankly, it is difficult to say how it affects sleep in pregnancy because there is already so much sleep disruption happening! However, this uncomfortable sensation in the legs, combined with the need to move them, may make it even harder for you to fall asleep.

Those women who have restless legs syndrome have an 80% chance of also having "periodic limb movement disorder." This occurs when one or both legs move repeatedly in a motion that involves the big toe flexing and the other toes fanning out. It can also involve flexing of the ankle, knee, and even the thigh. Usually it is just one leg moving at a time: one leg jumps or twitches for a while and later the other one may start up. These movements each last for 1–10 seconds and often continue at regular intervals of 20–40 seconds, during the light stages of sleep. They can cause mini-arousals in your sleep and occasionally they contribute to nighttime awakenings. However, usually they go unnoticed except perhaps by the person who shares the bed.

Snoring is also a frequent companion of pregnancy. By the third trimester about two-thirds of women are aware of snoring at least sometimes, and many have breathing irregularities during sleep. These irregularities are called "sleep disordered breathing." They can include loud snoring, shallow breathing, and/or partial or full obstruction of the upper airway during sleep. Airway obstruction can cause you to stop breathing for short periods called "apneas" (which literally means "without breath"). These breathing irregularities are especially likely to occur in late pregnancy and generally subside after the baby's birth, except in some women who already had sleep disordered breathing prior to pregnancy. Sleep disordered breathing can disrupt sleep, increase blood pressure, and affect cardiovascular health. Women who are overweight are especially prone to this type of breathing disorder during sleep. If you suspect that you have breathing irregularities during sleep, whether pregnant or not, you should tell your doctor.

So that's the bad news about sleep in pregnancy. The "up" side of the story is that some of the sleep disorders that arose during pregnancy subside after the baby's arrival. Now the baby himself or herself becomes the source of big-time sleep disruption!

WHAT HAPPENS TO SLEEP AT DELIVERY AND POSTPARTUM?

Childbirth is a time when your sleep is bound to be totally disrupted. Face it: Your sleep will be wrecked. For the hours around the actual birth, no one can predict when and how much sleep you will get. It will be influenced by your physical state, your emotional state, the duration of labor, the type of delivery, the time of the baby's arrival, prior sleep loss, how much excitement there is around you, and probably many other factors. Women just fall asleep when they can during this momentous experience.

The "postpartum" period is the time shortly after childbirth. Now there are two individuals—mother and infant—with sleep patterns that are intertwined, each affecting the other. During this time, the demands of feeding and care of the newborn disrupt the mother's sleep and her nighttime sleep is shorter than it was during pregnancy. However, the mother now takes more naps. Researchers from New Zealand looked at sleep patterns of women at 4 different weeks during pregnancy and postpartum. They found that women got the least sleep in the week immediately after delivery. In addition, during that week, 70% of women were napping 4 or more times per day. This was much higher than napping rates at the other times.

As in late pregnancy, the period after delivery is a time when some women have anxious dreams about their baby being in danger. It is not uncommon to have dreams of losing or forgetting about the baby. When awakening from such a dream, mothers may go to check on the infant to make sure everything is okay. Again, such dreams reflect normal concerns about the welfare of the child, and they may actually be adaptive in helping mothers to express and work through their anxieties about mothering.

The mother's sleep improves as the baby grows. At 3 months of age, the baby's sleep pattern becomes more regular and so does the mother's. And at some point, usually by 6 to 12 months, the baby will be sleeping through the night. Hurray! The mother's sleep generally improves but may not be as solid as it once was for some time—perhaps because she remains vigilant for the baby's cries at night.

Women who develop persistent insomnia sometimes identify childbirth as the starting point of their poor sleep. At my insomnia clinic, mothers of infants describe the enormous influence of their baby's sleep and wake patterns on their own. Often mothers will try to grab a few winks while their baby is sleeping, if they can. Surprisingly, there is little research on the *interaction* of baby and mother sleep. We do know that a mother's sleep is more likely to be disrupted than a father's. Researchers from the Netherlands found that a mother's insomnia was worse than the father's before childbirth and it remained worse over the first year after childbirth.

Rest or sleep when your baby sleeps. Forget about housework and other things that used to be important. Let the dishes pile up, and as my friend Helen says, "Let the dust bunnies gather dust." If you have other young children, it may be tricky, but try setting a naptime or quiet time for everyone, including yourself, so that everyone takes the same rest period. When you are up for nighttime feedings, keep visual, auditory, and tactile stimulation to a minimum. Importantly, keep the lights low and make the atmosphere quiet and subdued, so that both you and your baby can get back to sleep easily. Also, give yourself a pep talk: You can still function okay even though you are sleep deprived. This won't last forever; your baby will some day be sleeping through the night. All this is much easier if you have other adults to help you: someone to help during the daytime, and someone to do some, or all, of the nighttime feedings. Not everyone is so fortunate, but if you do have people who are willing to help, let them, so that you can get some sleep.[1]

WHAT HAPPENS AS YOUR CHILD GROWS OLDER?

It will be no surprise to you that as the baby grows and becomes a toddler and then a pre-schooler, that the mother's sleep continues to be influenced by her child's sleep. This relationship has seldom been researched, but one study did examine this issue using a survey. The results showed that the more disrupted the child's sleep, the poorer the mother's sleep was. Furthermore, mothers of children with sleep problems had a high number of child-related awakenings. Interestingly, the age of the child didn't matter: The mother's sleep was related to the child's sleep disruption whether the child was a preschooler or a pre-teen. Of course, if there are several children in the family, there is likely to be even more sleep disruption for the mother. In general, mothers continue to be responsive to their children at night and as a result, their own sleep continues to be affected by the children's sleep.

When children reach adolescence, it may not be their sleep problem that affects the mother's sleep so much as the late hours that the son or daughter keeps. Adolescents tend to have late bedtimes and late getting-up times, something called "phase delay." This phase delay in the biological clock, combined with teenage social activity, sometimes leads to the adolescent coming home late at night, after the parents are in bed. This can cause sleep disruption for the whole family, but perhaps especially for the mother who may be waiting up for the daughter or son to arrive home.

WHAT HAPPENS WHEN YOU ARE BUSY WORKING FOR A LIVING?

Ever lie in bed thinking about problems at work? A large survey of Swedish workers showed that almost one-quarter of women had sleep disruption at least once per week because of work-related thoughts. Studies have confirmed that being a woman, having high work demands, and not having input into work decisions are all associated with insomnia. On the other hand, having a supportive boss makes people less likely to have persistent insomnia. In general, you are more likely to have sleep problems if your job is demanding and you have little control, and when paid work and family life pull you in different directions. Since women frequently have demands on their time at work and at home, it's no wonder that so many of us have sleep problems.

---

[1]Thanks to Dr. Barbara Parker for sharing some practical tips for women during pregnancy and postpartum.

With economic uncertainties and financial cutbacks, restructuring of workplace organizations is another big source of stress. Such upheavals in our workplaces increase the risk of insomnia. And of course any kind of job insecurity is likely to affect sleep in a negative way.

For thoughts and concerns that keep you awake, try separating out the stressors that are within your control from the ones that are not. In the evening, at least 2 hours before bed, make a list of the concerns or issues that have been on your mind. Acknowledge the ones that are outside your control, and write "nothing for me to do tonight" beside them. For the stressors and issues that are within your control, decide which ones you will take on. Sometimes we have to pick our battles. Break the chosen ones into *very* small steps. Steps could involve actions like calling a friend for advice, checking the Internet to see who your Employee Assistance Program provider is, making an appointment to speak with your boss, and so on. Next, write down when you plan to do the first step; for example "tomorrow at noon." Then put your list "to bed" for the night. Place it in a drawer. Then when you are in bed and any issue from your list comes to mind, tell yourself you have dealt with it for the night. Then gently move your mind toward visual images. For example, imagine walking down your street and seeing your neighbors' homes and whatever else there is to be seen on your street.

THE BIG M: WHAT HAPPENS WHEN MENOPAUSE APPROACHES AND ARRIVES?

If you are approaching, have reached, or passed menopause, and your sleep is disrupted, you are not alone! At least half (estimates are 50%–80%) of women have sleep complaints during this time. When you think of how many women this represents in the population, the numbers are staggering. The prevalence of insomnia takes a steep rise at the time of the menopausal transition.

Menopause is the time when menstruation ceases permanently, medically defined when no periods have occurred for 1 year. This occurs around age 50. That is one specific point in time, so when we speak about going through menopause, what we usually mean is going through the "menopausal transition." This encompasses the time from the first signs of approaching menopause—when periods start becoming more irregular—all the way through to the time after menopause when symptoms like hot flashes are continuing to occur.

The most obvious physical experiences of the menopausal transition are hot flashes and sweating. About 75% of women will experience hot flashes. These usually go on for 1–2 years, sometimes for 5 years, and in 9% of women, for many years. It is these hot flashes, which occur most often at night, that frequently disrupt sleep. You may find it interesting that the arousal from sleep usually occurs just *before* the heat surge that comes with a hot flash, rather than vice versa. Our understanding of the exact causes of hot flashes is still sketchy. Altered levels of neurotransmitters (chemical messengers between nerve cells) in the brain, and falling levels of female hormones may lead to your internal thermostat being temporarily re-set. This results in a release of heat that can be very uncomfortable. A hot flash can be accompanied by significant sweating, palpitations (irregular heart beats), headaches, and nausea. It may be followed by shivering as the body's thermostat re-sets itself. Some women have to get up and change the sheets on the bed because of the intensity of the heat surge and the associated sweating. Whatever the exact mechanism and physiology of hot flashes, it is clear that many women have sleep disturbance in connection with them. Getting to sleep and staying asleep can both be problematic when hot flashes are happening.

If your sleep is interrupted by hot flashes, try keeping the bedroom cool, using fans, and making your bed in layers that can be peeled off and put back on as needed. If you have a bed partner, communicate during the day about your hot flashes and develop a system so you are not fighting about bed covers at night! Some medications may be helpful for severe hot flashes that are interfering with your life and sleep. Hormone replacement therapy (HRT), prescribed by your physician may be useful if it is started in the early stages of menopause. HRT involves taking a preparation of estrogen by itself or estrogen with progesterone. This is usually in the form of a pill, but is also available as a patch, gel, or vaginal ring. However, this treatment would only be started after a thorough discussion with your physician about the benefits and risks of this therapy as applied to you. Other medications that are sometimes helpful for reducing hot flashes are clonidine and selective serotonin reuptake inhibitors (SSRIs). These medications affect levels of adrenalin and serotonin, respectively, two neurotransmitters that are involved in hot flashes. Make sure you discuss any kind of medication decision with your physician and ask as many questions as you need to.

In studies of insomnia in women who had breast cancer, Dr. Josée Savard and her colleagues in Quebec City found that cognitive behavioral therapy for insomnia (CBT-I) worked well to improve sleep. Many of the participants had hot flashes, either because of naturally occurring menopause or premature menopause brought on by anti-estrogen cancer treatments. Dr. Savard observed that sleep improved with CBT-I, whether or not the woman had hot flashes at night (personal communication). This is evidence that CBT-I works to improve sleep for women who have hot flashes. My clinical experience tells me so as well. CBT-I can be used to reverse insomnia despite nighttime hot flashes.

Another thing that happens during the menopausal transition is that women become more and more likely to have sleep disordered breathing, that is, breathing irregularities during sleep. This often involves episodes of very shallow breathing through a partially obstructed airway, called "hypopneas" or "upper airway resistance." Sometimes, women will have repeated episodes of breathing cessation that last at least 10 seconds, called "apneas." When a woman passes menopause and enters the postmenopausal years, she is more likely than she was before to develop sleep disordered breathing, including "obstructive sleep apnea." The likelihood is probably at least 20%. All these types of breathing irregularities tend to disrupt sleep. Even if you are not waking up fully when the episodes occur, your sleep may be lighter and more disturbed. The typical symptoms that women experience when they have this type of breathing irregularity are loud snoring, morning headaches, daytime sleepiness, lack of energy, disrupted sleep, and sometimes depression. The higher prevalence of sleep disordered breathing in postmenopausal years is believed to be due to an increase in abdominal fat and the decrease in levels of the female hormone progesterone. Postmenopausal women who are overweight are especially likely to have disordered breathing during sleep.

See your physician if you suspect that you have any breathing irregularities during sleep. For example, if family members are telling you that your snoring is disturbing their sleep, if you think you may have stopped breathing for a time, if you have woken up gasping, short of breath, or with a big snore, these would raise your suspicion of a breathing issue. You should know that there are very effective treatments available for sleep disordered breathing. Your family doctor may decide to send you a sleep lab to see exactly what is happening overnight.

You may have heard of "CPAP" which stands for Continuous Positive Airway Pressure. This is the most common treatment for obstructive sleep apnea. CPAP is gentle air pressure applied through your nose and sometimes also through your mouth to prevent breathing obstructions in the upper airway. It involves wearing a "mask," or nasal "pillows," to deliver air while you sleep. The pressure of the air keeps your airway open. Don't be scared off by this! Many people so enjoy their new-found sleep with this equipment that they are very grateful for it. CPAP is not the only treatment. Depending on the nature and severity of your breathing problem, an oral appliance, like a mouth guard, may allow your airway to remain unobstructed during sleep. Many women have only mild obstructive sleep apnea, and depending on what the sleep lab study shows, "positional therapy" may be recommended. This is sleeping on your side, or with the head of the bed elevated. This strategy is sometimes enough to manage mild breathing problems overnight.

In addition to hot flashes and breathing irregularities, the other major aspect of a woman's experience that can interact with sleep is her mood. One study of women who were approaching menopause found that depressed mood, anxiety, and worrisome thoughts about not sleeping were all related to poor sleep. It is always difficult to tell which comes first when it comes to insomnia and mood. Distress and low mood can lead to poor sleep and vice versa. It's a circular relationship.

If you are having mood issues during the menopausal transition, there are some things that will help. First of all, know that you are not alone and you are not going crazy. Talk to other women to hear about their menopausal mood experiences. Talk to your physician so that he or she is aware of your mood and can assess whether you have a clinical depression. Two main treatment approaches work for depression. One is antidepressant medication. There are several categories of antidepressants and they are all about equally effective for mood. Each medication has its own set of potential side effects. Some antidepressants can make you sleepy and may be helpful for your sleep when taken at bedtime. If you are interested in trying antidepressant medication, then discuss this with your family physician. He or she will suggest an antidepressant to try and will probably follow-up with you again in a few weeks to see how it's working. The other approach is psychotherapy— or "talk therapy." Psychotherapies that have substantial research evidence to back their effectiveness for treating depression are cognitive behavioral therapy and interpersonal therapy. Ask your health care provider or consult your community resources to find a qualified, and preferably licensed, psychologist or therapist.

If you have anxious thoughts about not sleeping, see if you can pinpoint your main concerns and write them down during the daytime. Often they seem more extreme or catastrophic during a sleepless night than they are when we examine them in the daylight. See if you can bring them down to earth. Re-read relevant parts of Chapter 3 to reassure yourself if need be. Then, when you are in bed at night, you can remind yourself of your new, less extreme or worrisome sleep-related thoughts.

Of course, there may also be external sources of sleep disruption. Even if your children no longer live at home, there may be cats, dogs, grandchildren, and snoring bed partners. Caring for aging parents or an aging spouse, or caring for anyone with a disordered sleep schedule (e.g., a person with Alzheimer's disease) will also disrupt your sleep. Your own illness or pain syndrome can also contribute to poor sleep. See Chapter 20 on medical conditions and sleep.

WHAT HAPPENS AFTER RETIREMENT AND BEYOND?

Well, if some of your insomnia was work related, then retirement may bring you some relief. You may have fewer pressures on your time and mind, and you may be more relaxed. Operating against this positive aspect, unfortunately, is a general trend as we get older for our sleep to worsen. As we age, three main things happen to sleep: We wake up more often in the night, we get less deep sleep, and we wake up earlier. These occur to both women and men but in general, women seem to be more aware of, and bothered by, poor sleep. Some of the age-related changes are normal developmental changes including a reduction of neurons (nerve cells) and alterations in our biological sleep–wake control systems. In older adults, the internal circadian "clock" appears to be set earlier, making us more like "larks" rather than "night owls." For example, say when you were in your 30s and 40s, you went to bed at 11 p.m. and got up at 7 a.m. Over the years, you find yourself getting sleepier earlier and earlier until you may be going to bed at 8 p.m. and waking up for the day at 4 a.m. or earlier. This is quite common, and is really only a problem if this earlier sleep schedule does not fit with your preferred daytime routine. This "advanced" schedule that comes with aging does allow you to get up with (or before) the birds, but it gives you less time in the evening to do things with friends and family.

> If you want to stay awake later at night and to sleep later in the morning, put yourself under bright light in the evening and have relatively dim light in the morning. This pattern of light and dark exposure mimics a more westerly time zone (think Hawaii). Your internal sleep–wake clock will respond accordingly. You do not need a special light; being under any type of bright lamp or ceiling light in your home will do. To protect your eyes, do not look directly at the light. Be under the bright light for at least 30 minutes as late in the evening as you can. If there is still daylight in the evening after dinner, then take a stroll outside to get some natural brightness in the evening hours.

As we humans get older, we are also more prone to disruptions caused not just by insomnia, but by other sleep disorders. Restless legs syndrome is that uncomfortable creepy-crawly sensation in the legs that makes you want to move them, especially in the evening. This is very common as we get older, and it is more common in women than in men. The vast majority of people who have restless legs also have jumpy movements of their legs during sleep, called periodic limb movement disorder. However, you can have periodic limb movements without having restless legs; the prevalence of periodic limb movement disorder is high. It has been estimated that about 45% of people over age 65 have periodic limb movements during their sleep. The rates seem to be similar for men and women in this age group. These movements can lead to arousals from sleep, and feeling that your sleep is not restorative.

Sleep disordered breathing becomes much more common as we age. As mentioned, after the menopausal transition, women are more and more likely to develop irregular breathing patterns during sleep—both hypopneas and full apneas. Not all women develop sleep disordered breathing as they get older, but the rates are quite high. A study in a sample of people aged 65-95 years showed that 56% of the women had significant breathing disturbances during sleep. This was especially likely to happen to women who were overweight. Other associated medical conditions are high blood pressure and type 2 diabetes.

> If you are very sleepy during the day so that you are falling asleep in different situations (e.g., while reading, while being a passenger in a car, while

listening to someone talking), it is important that you let your physician know. There are many possible reasons for excessive sleepiness, and in most cases the underlying causes are treatable. If you are snoring, if you are aware that you have sometimes stop breathing during sleep, then you are high risk of having sleep disordered breathing and this definitely warrants a discussion with your physician.

Many medical disorders and pain conditions affect sleep (see Chapter 20). Also many medications affect sleep. Of course, as we get older, we are more and more likely to be taking medications. Many prescribed and over-the-counter medications affect sleep. Examples are: medications for high blood pressure, some decongestants, some heart medications (e.g., for rhythm disturbances), some antidepressants, methylphenidate, and other stimulants used for Attention Deficit Disorder, some asthma medications, corticosteroids like prednisone, pain medications containing caffeine, theophylline for asthma, nicotine patches used for smoking cessation, and thyroid medication at certain levels. Medications that can make your breathing worse at night include: morphine-type medication used for pain, anything that sedates you, including sleep medications and formulations containing alcohol.

Read medication labels and discuss any medication concerns, including effects on your sleep, with your physician and/or pharmacist. They will have recommendations about the dosage, the time of day that you take the medication, or alternative treatments. For over-the-counter medications, the exact same advice applies.

THE GOOD NEWS

Effective treatments are available for most sleep disorders. For insomnia, women make up the majority of volunteer participants in treatment studies. Subsequently, much of the research data on insomnia and insomnia treatments of all kinds are based on the experiences of women. We know what the best treatments are for improving sleep. At this time, the best approach is CBT-I, the Sleep Therapy approach used in this book. Although we are not yet sure if CBT-I can be helpful during pregnancy, postpartum, or during severe illness, we know that it works to reverse insomnia during most stages of life including young adulthood, midlife, and old age.

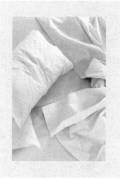

Chapter 19

You're a Man. Some Facts About Your Sleep

Although women tend to report insomnia in greater numbers, men have their share of sleep problems. So let's shine the spotlight on men's sleep now. Early discoveries about the nature of human sleep, and the effects of sleep deprivation, were largely based on research studies with male participants. For example, men comprised most of the volunteers in studies that revealed the existence of Rapid Eye Movement (REM) sleep in humans. In their landmark paper, published in the journal *Science* in 1953, Aserinsky and Kleitman, reported on "Regularly Occurring Periods of Eye Motility, and Concomitant Phenomena, during Sleep," that occurred in their 20 adult subjects, 18 of whom were men. Likewise, major advances in the understanding of our internal timekeeper and its relationship to sleep and wakefulness, were based on studies of men (and a few women) in time isolation, either in labs or in caves. A few brave men stayed in isolation in caves for months at a time to allow their physiological rhythms to be studied! Others subjected themselves to severe sleep restriction so that we could understand the effects of insufficient sleep on humans. These are just a few examples. Many men have volunteered in the name of sleep science, and at this point in history we know quite a lot about men's sleep.

TESTOSTERONE AND SLEEP

Testosterone, a hormone that occurs in much higher levels in men than in women, influences the development and maintenance of male sexual characteristics, including reproductive organs, body structure, beard growth, strength, sex drive, aggression, and mood. There are important connections between testosterone and sleep. Did you know that testosterone levels rise when you fall asleep? Levels continue to increase for about the first 90 minutes and then plateau, stay high during sleep and eventually peak around 8:00 a.m. They start to go down in the morning and continue to decline during the day reaching a low at around 8:00 p.m. This rhythm of testosterone depends on sleep; without sleep, testosterone does not show the normal nocturnal surge.

SLEEP-RELATED ERECTIONS

Erections during sleep, mainly in REM sleep, occur in healthy males from birth to old age. The average duration of a sleep-related erection is approximately 25 minutes. Because about 4 REM episodes occur over the night, the time spent per night in "penile tumescence" is around 90–100 minutes. As a man ages, the duration of these erections goes down slightly, but sleep-related erections and partial erections occur into very old age. Even though these events occur during REM sleep, the stage in which most of our dreaming occurs, they are unrelated to the content of dreams. Moreover, they have different physiological control mechanisms than do sexually stimulated erections during wakefulness. Nevertheless, problems with sexual erections ("erectile dysfunction") are sometimes assessed by measuring sleep-related erections; if erections are normal during sleep, then structural-mechanical problems are ruled out as a cause. The function of sleep-related erections remains a puzzle. Some have speculated that they provide regular, life-long practice and exercise for the erectile muscles and neural circuitry. This may have given our ancient male ancestors a reproductive advantage over other males who did not experience this phenomenon.

SEX AND SLEEP

Folklore has it that men fall asleep more quickly than women do after sex. Surprisingly, very little research has been done on this. You would think that we would know more about the normal interaction of sex and sleep—two activities that typically occur in the same place (the bed) at around the same time (at night). There is some evidence that men become quite sleepy after sex, and this may be connected with high levels of the hormones prolactin and oxytocin that occur after sexual intercourse. However, no scientific study has yet shown that men fall asleep faster than women after sex. It seems there are large differences among individuals—both men and women—in degree of sleepiness or alertness after sex. One study suggests that men, more so than women, think they fall asleep faster after sex, compared to no sex. Let's leave it at that.

SLEEP DISORDERS

Insomnia

When sleep is studied objectively, men's sleep usually looks worse that women's, but when asked about their sleep, men tend to have fewer complaints. Persistent, severe insomnia is reported by approximately 8%–10% of men. Even though this is lower than the insomnia prevalence reported by women, this represents a substantial number of men in the population. As in women, insomnia is more likely to occur when we have a medical disorder (e.g., diabetes, heart disease, chronic obstructive pulmonary disease), a pain condition (e.g., arthritic joints), and especially depression, stress, or other mental health challenges. Some studies suggest that men who maintain a healthy weight and those who are physically active are less likely to have insomnia. For anyone with persistent insomnia, as I've said in previous chapters, research shows that cognitive behavioral therapy for insomnia (CBT-I) is the treatment of choice. The vast majority of men do not get effective treatment for their insomnia, either because they don't seek help, or because CBT-I is not available in their community. So, here's your chance to reverse insomnia using the CBT-I based Sleep Therapy in this book. With a little bit of time and effort, you will be able to achieve satisfying sleep.

There are two sleep disorders that occur more frequently in men than in women. These are "sleep disordered breathing" and "REM sleep behaviour disorder." I'll outline what these are, in case they apply to you or someone you know.

Sleep Disordered Breathing

Two-thirds of men snore. What exactly is snoring? It is sound produced by vibration of structures in the upper airway, such as the soft palate, the uvula, and the walls of the pharynx (back of the throat). Basically, membranous structures in the upper airway that are not supported by cartilage can flutter and contribute to snoring. Sometimes snoring is mild and only a nuisance. On the other hand, loud snoring can be a sign of "obstructive sleep apnea." This is a sleep disorder in which people stop breathing (for periods of 10 seconds or more) during sleep, several times per hour. Each period of breathing cessation is called an "apnea." During an apnea, there is silence, which is broken by a loud snort as breathing resumes. If you have obstructive sleep apnea, you may be *un*aware of these breathing changes during the night. However, other people in your house may be aware, and your bed partner will certainly be aware.

Sleep professionals use the general term "sleep disordered breathing" to refer to obstructive sleep apnea and similar breathing problems that occur when the upper airway is partially or totally obstructed during sleep. The obstruction occurs when the muscles of the airway relax and collapse inward during sleep. Awakenings (often not remembered) happen many times per night as the body attempts to restore airflow. As a result, sleep is interrupted repetitively. The disrupted sleep makes the person very sleepy during the daytime. Sleep disordered breathing is three times more common in men than in women.

If you fall asleep easily much earlier than your normal bedtime, for example, in front of the television after dinner, and you struggle to stay awake at meetings or public events during the day, you may have excessive daytime sleepiness. Excessive daytime sleepiness, loud snoring, waking with snorts or gasping for air, and waking up with a headache are all possible symptoms of sleep disordered breathing and they warrant a trip to your family physician as soon as possible.

Being overweight increases the risk and severity of sleep disordered breathing. Another thing that makes sleep disordered breathing worse is alcohol—it makes apneas longer and more frequent. Some sedatives and sleeping pills, for example, the benzodiazepines, may have similar effects. Smoking can also make upper airway problems worse. So, to minimize your risk, maintain a healthy weight, minimize alcohol, avoid sedatives, and become a non-smoker if you aren't already. Alcohol and smoking are both difficult habits to quit and when you are ready, help is available. Relevant places to start would be your local health unit or your family physician.

An overnight stay in the sleep lab allows sleep disordered breathing to be assessed. In addition to monitoring your breathing, the assessment shows how your sleep is affected by any breathing irregularities. Because breathing stoppages can reduce the amount of oxygen in your blood, blood oxygen saturation is also measured overnight by a small sensor placed on the tip of a finger.

The treatment for sleep disordered breathing depends on the results of the sleep lab assessment and the recommendations of a sleep specialist. Treatments include positional therapy, weight loss, continuous positive airway pressure (CPAP), oral appliances, and in some cases, surgery such as tonsillectomy. With the correct treatment, the airway stays open all night, allowing you to breathe well and sleep well, and to be alert rather than sleepy during the daytime. As explained in the previous chapter on women's sleep, CPAP, one of the most common treatments, provides air pressure support for the airway to prevent it from collapsing, and it is very effective for obstructive sleep apnea. I have heard many men with sleep apnea report that CPAP improves their sleep and they feel so much better during the daytime.

Positional Therapy

I remember a nurse at the Toronto Western Hospital sleep lab, where I worked years ago, showing patients who had obstructive sleep apnea how to attach a sock containing a tennis ball to the back of their pajamas. It was usually done with a safety pin. This trick of the trade is still used today in order to prevent rolling onto one's back during sleep. If you do roll back, there is an immediate reminder—a firm nudge—to avoid this position. Positional therapy means sleeping in positions that minimize sleep disordered breathing. One of the best positions is on your side. Another option is to sleep with your head and trunk elevated by 30 to 60 degrees. However, this elevation is not easily achieved unless you have a hospital bed or another type of adjustable bed, or you arrange the pillows "just so." Sleeping on your side is probably the easiest solution.

REM Sleep Behavior Disorder

REM Sleep Behavior Disorder (RSBD) is not nearly so common as sleep disordered breathing, but at least 85% of diagnosed cases are in men over the age of 50. Big, sometimes violent, movements during REM (dreaming) sleep characterize this disorder. Normally in REM sleep, our muscles are relaxed and inhibited from moving. This prevents us from acting out our dreams. With this disorder, the muscles lose the normal inhibition in REM and people *do* act out their dreams! As you can imagine, this often leads to injuries to the dreamer and to anyone else nearby, especially the bed partner. So, if there is any chance you have RSBD, it is very important to seek medical help. If your family physician is not familiar with it, ask for a referral to a sleep lab.

EXERCISE AND SLEEP

My cousin Ted asked me, "The guys playing old timer hockey at 11 at night—is this good or bad for sleep?" It's a good question. First of all, as you've probably found, if you're wound up after a game, you need time to unwind (for example, by doing a crossword, watching television, or reading) before you go to bed. Otherwise you might be too stimulated to sleep. Second, the research indicates that *if you are already a good sleeper*, your sleep may be a few minutes longer after playing an active sport, compared to a night without such activity; you might even get a minute or two more of deep sleep. The changes are usually quite subtle. Third, if you have *insomnia*, playing a sport late at night will probably not help your sleep. It might even make it worse. For insomnia, your best bet is to exercise on a regular basis (not just the occasional pick-up game), for at least 30–45 minutes, several times (4-7) per week, in the afternoon or early evening. This may help you to fall asleep faster and to sleep longer. We don't know yet whether there is a "best" type of exercise for improving sleep when you have insomnia, but brisk walking, aerobics, and weight training have all been shown to be helpful. Combine regular exercise with CBT-I, and insomnia doesn't have much of a chance. This is just as true for women as for men.

AGING

With age, men's sleep, like women's, becomes shorter and more broken up by awakenings. So don't expect to get the same quality or quantity of sleep at age 60 as you did in your 20s. There are many contributors to these age-related sleep changes, discussed in Chapter 18. Testosterone production also declines with age; levels in the blood go down about 1%-2% per year from midlife onward. This may account for the slight decrease in duration of sleep-related erections with age. A number of physical changes occur over time that some have called "andropause." These changes are believed to result from declining testosterone levels, and they include decreased sexual desire and erectile quality, depression and fatigue, reduction in muscle and bone strength, increased fat, changes in skin and body hair, and altered sleep patterns. However, whether this is a clinical condition or just normal aging is debated, as is the use of testosterone replacement therapy for these changes. Testosterone treatment, or "androgen therapy," has potential risks that have not been fully studied in older men, so be sure you talk to your physician about the risks and benefits of this treatment if you are considering it. With respect to sleep specifically, it is not clear whether androgen therapy helps. We *do* know that low levels *and* high levels of testosterone are both connected with sleep disturbances. High doses of testosterone, when used illicitly (e.g., by some bodybuilders) can lead to significant sleep disturbance.

Some types of prostate cancer are treated with "androgen deprivation therapy," which is the opposite of androgen therapy. This is meant to reduce levels of testosterone in order to stop or slow the growth of prostate cancer cells. Several side effects can occur with this treatment, including weight gain, decreased muscle, breast development, loss of body hair, erectile dysfunction, decreased libido, increased emotionality, and hot flashes. Androgen deprivation is also associated with an elevated chance of having insomnia. Sex life can also be affected by all of this, but research indicates that after some adjustment to changes, some couples can adapt successfully and continue to enjoy sexual activity. Your physician can also help with advice on sexual aids, including medications; and some cancer clinics and other centers offer counseling to help restore sexual intimacy. Insomnia that occurs with cancer can be helped by CBT-I, the type of program used in this book. Sleep problems can occur with many other medical disorders and you will find more information in the next chapter.

WORK, TRAVEL, SPORTS, AND SLEEP

Work and travel schedules often put severe limitations on sleep. For example, professional hockey players not only have punishing physical requirements on the ice, but their schedules of home and away games are grueling. Playing games night after night, practices, and traveling to different time zones allow little time for rest and sufficient sleep. Insomnia becomes a problem and some players will take sleeping pills. The National Hockey League has a substance abuse and behavioral health program and there is now emphasis on ways to rest and sleep without sleep medication. Alex Burrows of the Vancouver Canucks was quoted as saying: "They've given us tricks to control our breathing, methods to help us sleep, whether it's iPhone apps or other things to lower your heart rate and allow you to get better sleep. It works." So, even extreme challenges to sleep that occur with work and travel schedules can respond to behavioural methods. They take more time and attention than popping a sleeping pill, but CBT-I methods are safer and much more effective in the long run.

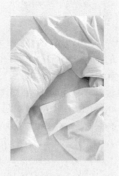

Chapter 20

You Have a Health Problem. Let's Talk About Your Sleep

If you are dealing with a health problem, chances are your sleep is also a problem. Surveys from all over the world show that people who have medical conditions are especially likely to have sleep problems. This book does not have space for every medical condition that exists, so I have selected a few conditions that are highly prevalent in North America, and those most often reported by people with insomnia. I hope that I have included the ones that you are most interested in.

The connection between medical conditions and sleep is a complex and circular one. A medical condition can lead to a sleep problem, and a sleep problem can lead to a medical condition. Each can exacerbate the other. There is a particularly strong link between chronic pain and sleep difficulty.

CHRONIC PAIN

Chronic pain is pain that has lasted for 6 months or longer. You will know if you have chronic pain. It will be your constant, difficult companion. Some examples of chronic pain conditions are fibromyalgia; chronic back, neck, shoulder, or leg pain; recurrent headaches; rheumatoid arthritis; osteoarthritis; and ankylosing spondylitis (a rheumatic disease involving inflammation of the joints in the spine). There are many others. Sometimes pain remains in our bodies after a car crash, sports injury, or other incident.

Most people with chronic pain have insomnia. Several research studies have shown that as pain intensifies, sleep gets worse, and as sleep gets worse, pain intensifies. You probably have noticed this connection. How to stop this cycle? You are most likely trying to manage the pain itself by trying to get comfortable at night through positioning your body in bed and/or using various means to manage the pain (exercise, medications, physiotherapy, and other helpful strategies). This may not be enough, however, to stop the cycle of pain and sleep disturbance. For this, I suggest cognitive behavioral therapy for insomnia (CBT-I). An important study, published in 2000, from Ottawa with people who had various chronic pain conditions including back pain, neck pain, leg pain, and pelvic pain, found that people's sleep improved very well with CBT-I. The participants were still sleeping well, and even longer still, when they were studied again 3 months later.

Subsequent studies have confirmed that CBT-I improves sleep in people who have chronic pain. This includes people with fibromyalgia and people with osteoarthritis. A study with older adults who had osteoarthritis showed that CBT-I worked very well to improve sleep and that sleep improvements were sustained 1 year later. It is particularly interesting that, in addition to improving sleep for the long-term, CBT-I can also improve pain control. So, if you have chronic pain and insomnia, CBT-I is an excellent technique to use. The CBT-I–based Sleep Therapy program in this book may help you replace a vicious cycle of pain and sleep disturbance with a positive cycle of better sleep and better pain management.

Some people ask me about exercise for improving sleep for people who have pain. The research results show that aerobic exercise—like walking, running, biking, aerobics, swimming, aquafit—reduces pain and fatigue, and improves fitness and quality of life. However, the direct effects on sleep are not so obvious. So, I definitely recommend aerobic exercise for chronic pain and for your overall health and well-being, but if you want to sleep well, add CBT-I.

If you are fortunate enough to be able to participate in a multidisciplinary chronic pain program that includes cognitive behavioral therapy for pain (this is different from CBT-I but it may involve some of the same components, like relaxation or meditation), this is often very helpful for pain management. These programs may also involve physiotherapy, occupational therapy, dietary advice, and information on pain and pain medications. I do recommend these programs. Whether they also improve sleep is not yet clear—some studies say "yes" and some say "no." It certainly will not make your sleep worse. If you want to be sure of improving your *sleep*, then CBT-I is what you want.

HEART DISEASE

Heart disease, or "coronary artery disease" occurs when there is a build-up of plaque on the walls of the arteries (vessels that supply blood) to your heart. This makes the arteries narrower and the heart may not get the blood flow and oxygen that it needs. This can lead to chest pain or "angina," shortness of breath and fatigue. Sometimes people don't have any symptoms and don't know that they have heart disease. If you wonder about your own risk of heart disease, ask your family physician about this and ask what you can do to reduce your risk of heart attack or stroke.

Carol experienced a heart attack at the age of 69. She was slim, athletic, and had a healthy diet. This event turned her world upside down. Carol was the last person anyone expected to have heart disease. She underwent coronary bypass surgery. While in the hospital she had great difficulty sleeping and she was given some sleep medication at night. When she left the hospital and started her cardiac rehabilitation program she found she could not sleep at home. Basically, she felt she had no control over her heart and was afraid of having another heart attack and dying during sleep. Now she had no control over her sleep. She decided to take the Sleep Therapy program, and slowly but surely, her sleep returned over 3 weeks. She started to sleep well again, without any sleeping pills. She gained confidence in her ability to sleep, and not only was her heart repairing itself, but she was reassured that her sleep system was strong and reliable.

If you have heart disease, the research indicates that you are especially likely to have insomnia, including trouble falling asleep, and waking up too early in the morning. There is also a higher-than-normal chance that you have some breathing irregularities during sleep. These irregularities are called "sleep disordered breathing." They can include loud snoring, shallow breathing, and/or partial or full obstruction of the upper airway during sleep. If you think you might have some breathing irregularities during sleep, it is important to see your physician as soon as possible. Treatment of these breathing problems can improve both your sleep and your heart health, including lowering your risk of heart attack.

Whether or not you have breathing irregularities at night, you probably have insomnia. Research shows that CBT-I, the techniques on which Sleep Therapy is based, improves sleep in people who have heart disease and insomnia. You might avoid staying up extremely late in case this puts extra stress on the heart, so when you are doing Sleep Therapy make sure that you don't limit your time in bed to less than 5 hours. People who have had heart disease have safely and successfully done all steps of the Sleep Therapy program in our clinic, and this is true for other clinics where people with various medical problems including heart disease have benefitted from CBT-I.

Some medications that are used for sleep can affect the heart and some depress breathing, so be sure to discuss the risks and benefits of any sleep medications with your physician and/or pharmacist. See Chapter 22 for more information on sleep medication.

CANCER

Cancer is not one disease but a large variety of diseases; each type is different from the others. What they all have in common is that there is an overgrowth of certain cells. The particular cell type that starts multiplying too fast determines the symptoms, the diagnosis, and where in the body the cells are most likely to spread. The treatment for the cancer depends on what type and stage of cancer it is. The most common types of cancer treatments are surgery, radiation, and chemotherapy.

Many people who have had cancer have sleep problems. Although sleep problems have not been studied in all types of cancer, they have been studied in lung, prostate, breast, colorectal, and head and neck cancers. People with lung cancer and women with breast cancer are especially likely to experience sleep difficulty. Let's talk about the types of sleep problems that are common and what to do about them.

If you have insomnia, you are not alone. Almost one-third of people attending our cancer center have insomnia. There are many reasons why insomnia often precedes, accompanies, and/or follows a cancer diagnosis. The most common contributors are thoughts and concerns—about one's health, family and friends, and the future. It is not unusual to be anxious, worried, and to feel discouraged or depressed in response to a cancer diagnosis. There is often uncertainty about what's next, fear of unfamiliar circumstances and treatments, and disruption of one's normal routine. Understandably, this emotional upheaval can contribute to insomnia. Younger people who receive a cancer diagnosis are especially likely to be distressed and to have sleep difficulty. The physical and mental stress of some treatments for cancer can also lead to sleep problems. People who have had recent cancer surgery are especially prone to insomnia; we are not sure exactly why, but it may have something to do with staying in the hospital, which is disruptive to sleep. The insomnia that occurs with cancer is, more often than not, accompanied by fatigue and exhaustion.

Sometimes physicians will prescribe sleep medication for short-term use when you have cancer. This can be very effective while you are dealing with the stress of the diagnosis and treatment. For the longer term, other options are more helpful. There is now a lot of evidence that CBT-I works well to help people who have had cancer. The same techniques that are in this book benefit people with cancer. Because it takes extra energy to carry out some aspects of Sleep Therapy, you will probably choose to do it after you have recovered from cancer treatments that sap your energy. With Sleep Therapy, people with cancer who have insomnia are sleeping well by the end of the program; their fatigue decreases, and they are functioning better during the daytime.

> When you start Sleep Therapy, take advantage of the afternoon nap if you are sleepy. As I described in Chapter 9, the prime nap zone is 1–4 p.m. Try to limit your nap to no more than an hour so that you are sleepy again by bedtime.

Some other types of interventions for cancer patients are being studied for their potential benefit to sleep. Some studies of relaxation techniques, Tibetan yoga, and exercise (such as walking) have shown improvements in sleep. However, these interventions for cancer patients have not yet been as carefully or extensively studied as has CBT-I.

Another common sleep problem for people who have had cancer is "restless legs." Restless legs occur while you are resting in the evening and you must move around to deal with a crawling, tingling, numb, or uncomfortable sensation in the legs. It usually goes away when you stretch or walk around. In a survey done at our cancer center, this was the most common sleep-related problem reported by patients: 41% of people said they had restlessness in their legs. We are not yet sure why this number is so high. Stretching and moving around is how most people deal with this leg restlessness, and some people find a warm bath before bed to be helpful. About 80% of people who have restless legs syndrome also have periodic limb movements (repetitive arm or leg twitches or jerks) during sleep. People are usually unaware of these, but their bed partner may notice them. Such movements can cause mini-arousals in your sleep. If you are very bothered by restless legs, I suggest that you tell your family physician. There are medications that can be prescribed to help reduce the interference of these leg sensations and/or limb movements with your sleep.

SEASONAL ALLERGIES

Many people have seasonal allergies—stuffy, running nose, and other symptoms in reaction to pollens or grasses. Naturally, it is difficult to get to sleep at night when your nose is congested. You may also be waking up during the night with a stuffy nose and finding it hard to breathe. Research shows us that nasal congestion is at its worst in the latter part of sleep—the early morning hours. People who experience seasonal allergies are more likely to snore and to have sleep disordered breathing (irregular, obstructed breathing), sometimes even sleep apnea (stopping breathing for short periods of time during sleep). These breathing irregularities are believed to be due mainly to nasal congestion. Your physician can prescribe medication (for example, corticosteroid nasal spray) for the nasal congestion and this, in turn, helps people to get a better sleep. You should avoid taking types of antihistamines that cause sleepiness, like some cold and flu medications for nighttime symptoms, because these can leave you feeling sleepy during the day, and you are probably already tired and sleepy because of disrupted sleep. It's best to talk to your physician or pharmacist about the options.

BEING OVERWEIGHT

If you are overweight, I'm sure you are aware of the many health benefits that come with losing weight. In terms of your sleep specifically, some very interesting relationships have been found between duration of sleep and weight. Shorter sleepers tend to have a higher body mass index and to gain more weight over time. In addition, short sleep and poor quality sleep seem to alter glucose metabolism (the way your body uses sugar) and may increase your risk of type 2 diabetes. Research also shows that short sleep is linked to appetite stimulation: It boosts levels of an appetite-stimulating hormone called ghrelin, and reduces levels of an appetite-suppressing hormone called leptin. We do not yet know what causes what, but there are strong connections between short sleep and being heavier and less healthy. I should point out right away that short sleep is *not* the same thing as insomnia (although you can have both). Short sleep usually occurs when people repetitively curtail their sleep because of their busy life, or it can occur naturally in people who don't need much sleep. So, the message is make time for sleep, because curtailing sleep may affect your metabolism and hinder weight loss.[1]

If you are overweight you are also at higher risk of having sleep disordered breathing. If you suspect you may be stopping breathing during sleep (or someone has observed this), then talk to your family physician as soon as possible. Other signs of breathing-related problems at night include being sleepy—you fall asleep quickly any time you have the chance—and loud snoring. These are indications that you need to get this checked. If you *do* discover that you have sleep apnea or other sleep disordered breathing problems, there are very effective treatments that will help you sleep more continuously during the night and reduce your daytime sleepiness.

DIGESTIVE DISCOMFORT

If you are prone to having heartburn (gastroesophageal reflux disease or GERD) at night, chances are you also have some sleep difficulty. This nighttime heartburn is sometimes accompanied by acid reflux and a cough. In large studies, people who have these symptoms are very likely to have disturbed sleep, and people who have insomnia are likewise prone to GERD. Some experts believe that GERD and insomnia each make the other worse, forming a vicious cycle. There are medications that can be prescribed by your physician to reduce GERD at night, and once the GERD is better, the research shows that sleep improves as well. If you still have some insomnia after the GERD is treated, and if there are no other major medical issues to deal with, then you can always use CBT-I, the Sleep Therapy program in this book, to deal with the unresolved insomnia.

People with bowel problems are also prone to sleep disturbance. Ulcerative colitis and Crohn's disease are types of inflammatory bowel disease, conditions that involve inflammation of the small and large intestine. The inflammation can bring abdominal pain, diarrhea, cramps, rectal bleeding, weight loss, and other symptoms. Irritable bowel syndrome, although not accompanied by inflammation of the bowel, occurs with diarrhea, and/or constipation and recurrent abdominal pain. Compared to people without bowel problems, people with inflammatory bowel disease and people with irritable bowel syndrome describe poorer sleep—taking a long time to get to sleep and waking up several times at night—and have greater fatigue. It is not yet clear why sleep laboratory studies do not pick up differences in sleep between people with bowel disorders and "normal" control participants. It is possible that the laboratory measures are somehow not capturing aspects of the sleep experience of the people with these disorders. People with these bowel disorders do report that when their bowel problem flares up, their sleep becomes worse and when their sleep is poor, they are more likely to have a flare-up of the illness. There are many types of medical and lifestyle treatments for these diseases. It makes sense that when the bowel condition is stable, sleep is bound to be better; and conversely, getting a good night's sleep can only

[1]If you are overweight and you have insomnia, it is okay to shorten your time in bed as part of Sleep Therapy because this will be temporary, and will allow you to have optimal sleep in the long run.

be helpful for the bowel condition. We do not know if CBT-I is effective in treating insomnia for people who have these conditions, because it has not yet been tested. I would think that if your bowel disorder is not severe, you would be very likely to benefit from CBT-I.

BREATHING PROBLEMS

When we move from wakefulness to sleep, our breathing rate decreases, and the flow of air in and out of the lungs is reduced. These sleep-related changes are more pronounced when we have a breathing problem: Our breathing becomes very difficult. You may have noticed this when you had a cold with a cough. You wake up a lot with coughing, especially toward the end of sleep. Many people with asthma find that it gets worse at night. There may be more coughing and wheezing, which are associated with awakenings and shortened sleep. In general, if breathing is difficult for any reason, then our sleep will be disrupted. This type of thing happens on a nightly basis when people have chronic breathing problems like emphysema (damage to the lungs) and chronic bronchitis (irritated bronchi that leads to coughing up sputum). Chronic obstructive pulmonary disease (COPD) is a term that encompasses emphysema and chronic bronchitis.

People with COPD often get very little sleep, and what they do get is disrupted. Their breathing problems get worse at night, especially during REM (dreaming) sleep, and sometimes the amount of oxygen in their bloodstream drops, and this can be a concern because our cells require sufficient oxygen to function properly. It is not uncommon for people with COPD to also have obstructive sleep apnea (breathing stoppages for short periods during sleep). This creates what's called "overlap syndrome" and the reduction of oxygen in the bloodstream can be severe when these two conditions occur together. Fortunately, there are various treatments for these problems and your physician can help here. There are also some techniques to manage shortness of breath that include "pursed lip breathing"—inhaling through your nose and exhaling as if blowing into a straw. A nurse who knows about COPD can provide information and show you these techniques. Apart from breathing problems, insomnia itself is also common when you have COPD, especially if you are anxious or depressed. It is best to avoid sleeping pills because they can make breathing more shallow. Research shows that CBT-I works well for insomnia when you have COPD.

KIDNEY DISEASE

People with kidney disease that has progressed to the point that they require dialysis have a very high rate of sleep disorders—insomnia, excessive daytime sleepiness, sleep apnea, and/or periodic limb movement disorder. Most have a combination of these. Up to 80% of people who have advanced kidney disease have restless legs syndrome. Sleep tends to be short and fragmented. Sleep disturbance and kidney disease seem to follow similar courses—they tend to worsen together. For insomnia itself, some researchers from Taiwan have found that the same type of program that I have described in this book (CBT-I) improved the sleep of people with kidney disease who were receiving periotoneal dialysis or hemodialysis. The patients' fatigue levels also improved. These early research findings lead me to believe that the program in this book should be appropriate and helpful for people with kidney disease. For other sleep disorders that people with kidney disease often have to deal with—restless legs, periodic limb movement disorder, and sleep apnea—your physician is the person to turn to for help.

NEUROLOGICAL DISORDERS

I will summarize some the findings about sleep when you, or someone you know, has Alzheimer's disease, Parkinson's disease, or multiple sclerosis.

Alzheimer's Disease

Sleep disturbances occur in about 40% of people with Alzheimer's disease. It is common for people to wake several times and for long periods at night. This is when wandering can occur. People with Alzheimer's disease seem to have an accelerated aging of their sleep control systems in the brain, so that they get less and less sleep at night, and tend to take more naps during the daytime. Sleep studies show that they get only low amounts of deep sleep and REM (dreaming) sleep. People with Alzheimer's need assistance to use sleep improvement strategies. Studies have shown that some of the CBT-I techniques, like having a constant rise time, and limiting naps are helpful. The full CBT-I program has not been systematically studied in people with Alzheimer's disease, probably because it is not feasible for caregivers to add this to all the other tasks they are attending to. Other strategies that have been helpful for sleep in people with Alzheimer's disease are exercise such as walking, and increased light exposure.

If you think the sleep of people with Alzheimer's disease is poor, you should ask caregivers of people with Alzheimer's how *they* sleep. Having to be alert during the day and at night, and the strenuous mental and physical activities required for Alzheimer's disease care, make for very poor sleep. In addition, family caregivers may have worries, depression, and reduction in pleasurable activities and in contact with friends. There is fear about what the future will bring, and huge anxiety around decisions about placing the person in care. As an estimate, 60%–70% of caregivers have sleep disturbances. Having a break ("respite care") to be able to have an afternoon nap, to do some exercise, and to see friends is very helpful for caregivers. We do not know yet whether respite care helps the caregiver's nighttime sleep specifically, and I have not yet seen any studies of CBT-I for caregivers of Alzheimer's patients. However, CBT-I for other caregivers *has* been studied; for example, it has been studied in family caregivers of people with cancer where it was found to be effective for improving sleep quality and increasing sleep duration.

Parkinson's Disease

Sleep difficulties, including frequent awakenings, and daytime sleepiness are very common for people who have Parkinson's disease. As the disease progresses, the sleep disturbance gets worse. In addition, people with Parkinson's disease are more likely than the general population to have some abnormalities in REM sleep, the sleep stage where we do most of our dreaming. Not everyone with Parkinson's has REM abnormalities. However, something called REM Sleep Behavior Disorder (RSBD), which involves moving around during REM sleep, is more likely to occur in people with Parkinson's disease than in the general population. We are not quite sure why. Normally movements are inhibited in REM so that we don't act out our dreams. People with RSBD lose some of this inhibition of movement and may act out their dreams, for example hitting and kicking, which leads to collisions with furniture and walls, and injuries to themselves and their bed partners. RSBD is usually treated with medication. As for insomnia, I have not seen any studies of CBT-I for people with Parkinson's disease. I expect that the principles and strategies of CBT-I (Sleep Therapy) would be helpful for people with Parkinson's disease, unless the disease is very advanced.

Multiple Sclerosis

Research suggests that at least half of people who have multiple sclerosis have insomnia. The most common reasons given by people for their insomnia are having to get up to urinate, pain and discomfort, and having a racing mind. Also, more people with the disease report breathing difficulties during sleep than do people in the general population. Fatigue and daytime sleepiness can also be significant problems. I have not seen any studies that looked at whether CBT-I can improve the sleep of people with multiple sclerosis who have insomnia. I would expect it to be helpful, at least for people whose disease is in remission, and for those with enough energy to carry out the CBT-I strategies.

IS CBT-I ALWAYS HELPFUL WHEN WE HAVE MEDICAL PROBLEMS?

A member of my family, Alec, was 92 years old when various health problems started to limit his social and active lifestyle. He was dealing with congestive heart failure, which caused his legs to swell, and his kidneys started to fail. He was having a very hard time sleeping. His doctor prescribed low dose trazodone for his sleep, which he took each night, but it did not really help. Even though his sleep was a big issue for him, I did *not* offer to show him Sleep Therapy techniques. He had very little energy and strength, needed oxygen from a tank, and assistance from a nurse to get into bed at night. This was not the time for him to be using Sleep Therapy techniques that involve getting out of bed when you are not sleeping, staying up to certain bedtimes, and keeping sleep diaries. This situation illustrates that CBT-I or Sleep Therapy is not always appropriate for people with medical conditions.

I believe that it is not so much the type of medical condition that limits how useful the techniques are, but rather the overall energy and strength of the person to carry out CBT-I. The usefulness of the techniques also depends on the person's interest in sleeping well and in using behavioral (nondrug) strategies to do so. To sum up, even though CBT-I has not yet been tested with all medical conditions, it probably works well to reverse insomnia regardless of the presence of medical conditions *if* you have the energy, strength, and motivation to do it.

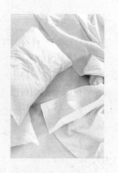

Chapter 21

You're Depressed or Anxious. Let's Talk About Your Sleep

Sadness and anxiety are normal human emotions. When we're feeling somewhat down or anxious, we can benefit from exercise (a wonderful natural antidepressant and stress buster), relaxation, recreation, eating nutritious foods, allowing time for sleep, and talking to a friend. However, when the sadness continues or the anxiety mounts to the point that our ability to do our usual activities is challenged, these are clinical conditions and we will benefit from professional help in addition to the self-care strategies just mentioned.

In cutbacks and restructuring at her workplace, Marie had lost her job as an account manager, a position she had held for 7 years. Prior to this blow, she had been feeling considerable tension at work, as she and her coworkers faced uncertainties about the looming changes. She received some severance pay but this would not last more than a few weeks; she didn't know how she was going to continue to pay the rent and to support her 2 teenagers. When she left work on the last day, Marie felt like taking refuge at home. She just wanted the world to go away and her problems to solve themselves. She went to bed and stayed there, under the covers. She didn't feel like getting up in the morning, nor the next morning. The shock and disappointment of losing her job turned into depression. Marie's mood was low and she couldn't see how things could improve in the future. The more she stayed at home, the harder it was to get out of the house. She started to feel vulnerable and panicky just thinking about going to the grocery store. As you can imagine, Marie's sleep was not good. She was unable to fall asleep, she was waking up during the night (sometimes in a panic), and she was waking up much earlier in the morning than she wanted to. Needless to say the sleep difficulty did not help her situation. It only made her feel more distressed, fatigued, and discouraged.

Unfortunately Marie's situation is not unique. Clinical depression and anxiety are very common conditions. Let's look at what they are, what happens to sleep, and what helps recovery of mood and sleep.

DEPRESSION

Depression often, but not always, begins with a loss or sudden change in the course of one's life. It's natural to feel sadness, anger, and discouragement when things go wrong, but when the blow is very big or extended over time, and/or we are particularly vulnerable to feeling low, the sadness can persist and develop into depression. Symptoms vary from person to person but depression involves low mood or a loss of interest in things that normally are pleasurable. It can also involve difficulty concentrating and making decisions, decreased (or sometimes increased) appetite, fatigue, self-blame, feeling discouraged, moving and thinking more slowly than usual, feeling agitated, having sleep difficulty, and having thoughts about death and suicide. If several of these symptoms continue every day for more than 2 weeks, this is what's called "clinical depression." If you think you may have clinical depression, it is important to get help as soon as you can. Start with your family physician or mental health professional; make an appointment to see him or her and discuss options for treatment. The degree of depression can range from mild to severe. In severe cases, people become quite hopeless, and getting help is imperative. It is difficult to help yourself when you are feeling so low.

Insomnia usually goes along with depression. In general, when we are depressed, we may take longer to fall asleep, wake up more during the night, and/or wake up too early in the morning. Sleep lab studies show some changes in Rapid Eye Movement (REM) sleep: It tends to start earlier in the night, and there's more than usual in the first part of the night. The amount of deep sleep is usually reduced. With some types of depression, a different pattern occurs—one of *hyper*somnia (excessive sleep). For example, with Seasonal Affective Disorder, which is depression that occurs with winter darkness and lifts with longer hours of daylight, people often sleep more than usual and have trouble waking up in the morning.

Depression and Insomnia: What Comes First?

Did you know that insomnia increases a person's risk of developing depression? Physicians and psychologists used to think that insomnia was part and parcel of a person's depression, that the insomnia came with the depression. However, now we know that insomnia often *precedes* depression. Over the last 25 years, many studies have followed people with insomnia over time. At least 20 of these have specifically looked at people's sleep and mood over *years*. These studies find that, compared to people without insomnia, people with insomnia have twice the risk of developing depression 1 or more years later. That's one of the reasons it is important to treat insomnia early; in doing so it may prevent the onset of depression.

It used to be thought that if you had both depression and insomnia, you needed to fix the depression and the insomnia would take care of itself. We now know that insomnia does not necessarily go away on its own, even when the depression lifts. We also know that it makes good sense to treat both conditions and not to delay either type of treatment.

How to Sleep When You're Depressed

I'll outline here what we know about treating insomnia in three forms of clinical depression: major depression (medically classified as Major Depressive Disorder), Seasonal Affective Disorder, and Bipolar Disorder.

Major depression

This is the most common type of clinical depression. First of all, it is wise to get help for the depression itself. The two most effective treatment approaches are antidepressant medication and psychotherapy. You can do one, do the other, or do them both. Antidepressant medications are usually prescribed by your family physician or a psychiatrist, who will base his or her recommendations and prescription on your specific symptoms and medical background. Typically, the physician will explain the benefits and side effects of the medication, outline how long the medication typically takes to work, and suggest that you return to follow-up within a few weeks.

Psychotherapy is talking with a counselor or therapist. I recommend a psychologist or other mental health professional who is trained in techniques that are "evidence-based," that is, they have been proven to work. Cognitive behavior therapy (CBT) is the most common evidence-based intervention for depression. CBT has a similar name to cognitive behavioral therapy for insomnia (CBT-I) and both involve cognitive (thinking) and behavioral (doing) techniques, but the two interventions are distinct. For depression that is severe, antidepressant medication is often recommended as the first treatment. The antidepressant medication may allow you to gain a bit of energy and concentration; then you will be more able to engage with your support network and in psychotherapy if you wish.

Guess what? If you are depressed and you also have insomnia, research shows that CBT-I works to help your sleep just as well as it works for people who are not depressed. Moreover, recent studies suggest that, not only does sleep improve, but mood improves too! For example, a study from Stanford University showed that participants' sleep improved, and also that half of them were no longer depressed after CBT-I. These are early results and more research is needed, but CBT-I is a very promising technique for people with insomnia and depression because it improves sleep and it seems to improve mood too, even though mood is not a specific focus of the techniques. These studies were done with people whose depression was *not* severe. For severe depression, it still makes sense to get medical help for the depression as the first and most important step in feeling better.

Seasonal affective disorder

As I mentioned earlier, with seasonal affective disorder, the sleep problem is usually hypersomnia, at least in the dark months, rather than insomnia. The wanting-to-stay-in-bed-in-the-morning feeling that occurs in the dark months with seasonal affective disorder appears to be linked to a delay of certain circadian rhythms, including melatonin, cortisol, and sleep–wake tendency. For this, bright light treatment (usually taken in the early morning) can help lift mood and reduce the hypersomnia. The timing and details of this treatment are very specific. Professionals with training in behavioral sleep medicine and/or circadian rhythm interventions can provide specific advice for your situation if you have seasonal affective disorder. Start by asking your family physician.

Bipolar disorder

Bipolar disorder is a certain type of mood disorder in which there are depressive episodes and also, less frequently, episodes of elevated (or sometimes irritable) mood during which the person has lots of energy, has grandiose ideas, and may engage in exciting and risky behaviors (e.g., over-spending, making ambitious plans, overindulging in alcohol or sex). Depending on how disruptive these episodes are to the person's life, they are either called "manic" (severe) or "hypomanic" (less severe). During the depressive episodes, sleep is similar to that of people with regular clinical depression. During the manic/hypomanic episodes, sleep–wake patterns are altered significantly. The person may stay awake for many hours past their usual bedtime, or even all night, because they are absorbed in a project or doing something interesting. Sleep is not very long and not very deep. REM sleep may occur earlier in the night, and there may be more of it than usual. Bipolar disorder is usually treated with medication by psychiatrists and/or family physicians. If mood and symptoms are well managed by medication then insomnia is less of a problem. CBT-I is *not* recommended for insomnia that occurs with bipolar disorder—in either the depressed or the manic phases. This is because it has not been adequately tested in this condition, and, more importantly, there is a small risk of triggering a manic episode with sleep deprivation, and CBT-I does involve a type of controlled sleep deprivation when you stay up later than your usual bedtime. Techniques for relaxing the body and the mind, for example, those in the chapter "What to Do With Your Mind" should be safe to use.

ANXIETY

Feeling anxious is a normal human experience. Anxiety serves some useful purposes: It can direct our attention and energy to important tasks and it can help us deal with threats to our safety. The latter is achieved via the "fight-or-flight" response—a surge of the hormones adrenalin and cortisol, with a sudden increase in heart rate, breathing, and many other physiological changes—that allow us to have strength and energy to fight or to run away from danger. You may have heard stories of super-human feats performed by people in catastrophic emergencies, such as lifting a car off a child who has just been hit, or plunging into raging waters to save someone who's drowning. This is when that adrenalin rush plays a crucial role. However, when our anxiety gets away from us, and its level exceeds what the situation calls for, for example, when we panic and we are not facing a life-threatening situation, then it can interfere with our well-being and functioning, and can be very uncomfortable. This is what is called "clinical anxiety."

There are several types of clinical anxiety; it is usually classified according to the types of symptoms that occur and/or the types of situations that provoke anxiety or fear. Examples are generalized anxiety, social anxiety, panic attacks, obsessions and compulsions, specific phobias, and posttraumatic stress. The following is some general information; your physician or psychologist can provide specific diagnosis and treatment if you think you have clinical anxiety. The main approaches to the treatment of the anxiety itself are psychotherapy and/or medication. For psychotherapy, I recommend an evidence-based treatment (i.e., a treatment that has been proven to work through research) that is specific to the type of anxiety that you have. For example, CBT including "exposure" techniques is often effective. "Exposure" is putting yourself in situations that make you anxious, starting with low-anxiety situations and working your way up to higher-anxiety situations while using strategies to relax and to manage your symptoms. The experience of being able to tolerate the once-avoided situation goes a long way to reducing the anxiety. For medication advice, consult your physician. Certain types of antidepressants or sedatives (benzodiazepines) are sometimes prescribed. Anti-anxiety medications have pros and cons, which you should definitely discuss with your physician.

Most people who have clinical anxiety also have insomnia: trouble falling asleep and/or trouble staying asleep. A common experience is having a racing mind when all you want is to fall asleep.

How to Sleep When You're Anxious

Most types of anxiety involve "hyperarousal"—the body and mind are on high alert. So, it's not surprising that sleep difficulties accompany anxiety. Discovering how to reduce that hyperarousal can be one key to reducing the sleep problem. Relaxation techniques can help with this (see Chapter 16). When a pattern of hyperarousal and sleep disturbance has continued over time, then new sleep patterns need to be established. This is when the Sleep Therapy (CBT-I) strategies of uncovering your natural sleep processes and associating your bed with sleep come in. However, as we'll see, severely restricting your time in bed as part of CBT-I may not be a good idea when you are prone to panic attacks, and we don't know yet whether CBT-I works if you have Obsessive-Compulsive Disorder. For most types of anxiety, though, CBT-I seems to work very well to improve sleep.

Generalized anxiety and social anxiety

Generalized anxiety is excessive anxiety and worry that is difficult to control, about a variety of issues such as events at work, family matters, your health and anything else that is happening. Social anxiety is discomfort and fear of being watched and judged by others, really not wanting to be the focus of attention, and avoiding such situations (e.g., by not volunteering to give talks, or not going to parties unless you are helping in the kitchen). For insomnia that occurs with these types of anxiety, CBT-I is probably helpful. I say "probably" because there have been very few proper research trials, but a few clinical studies of CBT-I suggest that people with elevated anxiety do just as well as anyone else at improving their sleep. So, the techniques in this book should be helpful. The chapter on "What to Do With Your Mind" will be especially helpful for dealing with nighttime worries and racing thoughts.

Panic attacks

Panic attacks are alarming anxiety episodes that come out of the blue. They are discrete periods of intense fear with physical symptoms that can include sweating, pounding heart, feeling short of breath, trembling, chest pain, nausea, dizziness, fear of losing control or dying, tingling, hot flashes or chills. The first time it happens, people can think they're having a heart attack. Sometimes panic attacks occur during sleep. These "nocturnal panic attacks" are sudden awakenings with fear, shortness of breath, rapid heart rate, and sweating. They are not associated with dreams, and from sleep lab studies we know that they do *not* occur in Rapid Eye Movement (REM) sleep. Rather, they occur in sleep Stages 2 or 3, often at the transition from Stage 2 to Stage 3 when breathing starts to slow down (see Appendix A for a description of sleep stages). Sometimes people develop insomnia because they are afraid to go to sleep and have another panic attack.

To my knowledge, no studies of CBT-I have been done specifically with people who have panic attacks. If you have daytime or nighttime panic attacks, you will benefit from learning more about them and knowing how to deal with the frightening physical alarm signals that occur with panic. The more you know what panic attacks are, and use strategies like deep breathing and self-reassurance, the more they will subside. This is best done with professional help, for example with evidence-based therapies that involve cognitive, behavioral, and exposure strategies, specifically for panic. Once you are comfortable with dealing with the panic attacks, and they subside, your sleep may improve substantially.

If it doesn't—your panic attacks are well managed but you still have insomnia—then CBT-I would be reasonable to try. You should know that there is a chance that sleep deprivation may bring on panic attacks, so you will want to avoid severely limiting your time in bed, unless you want more exposure practice.

Obsessions and compulsions

You may have heard of Obsessive-Compulsive Disorder (OCD). People with OCD have obsessions or compulsions or both. Obsessions are intrusive, anxiety-provoking thoughts that keep occurring even though you don't want them. Compulsions are repetitive behaviors or mental activity that are done to reduce anxiety, often in response to obsessions. For example, if a thought kept coming to mind again and again that you might set the house on fire (an obsession), this would naturally be very upsetting and frightening. You might take all sorts of precautions to make sure that the house does not catch on fire. For example, instead of checking that the stove is off and the toaster is unplugged once or twice, you would check them again and again, because of an uneasy feeling about them possibly being on. Again, for a specific diagnosis and treatment, seek help from your family physician or a psychologist.

If you have OCD and you have insomnia, no one knows for sure whether your insomnia will benefit from CBT-I because it hasn't been studied yet. Until we know, I would focus on managing your obsessive-compulsive symptoms with medication prescribed by your physician, and/or evidence-based methods with a psychologist or other professional. My clinical experience tells me that is difficult to benefit from CBT-I if OCD is severe, that is, if you are spending several hours each day being bothered by obsessions and/or compulsions. If the OCD is mild and/or well-controlled by medication, and insomnia remains an issue, then CBT-I *may* be helpful.

> I once saw a young man, we'll call George, who had OCD symptoms focused on his insomnia problem, and his mind was always trying to fix the problem and control his sleep. He was determined not to use prescribed medications for OCD or for insomnia. He had tried many techniques and herbal remedies for insomnia. When he tried CBT-I, unfortunately his obsessions prevented him from letting go and trusting his innate rhythms of sleep and wakefulness to work for him. His overactive mind, trying to control things, got in the way. His sleep did not improve substantially with CBT-I. I have a hunch that if George had been open to taking medication prescribed by his family doctor for OCD, this may have reduced the obsessions enough to allow him to benefit from CBT-I.

Specific phobias

A "specific phobia" is a fear of certain things like snakes, heights, or riding in elevators. No research is available on whether CBT-I is helpful for insomnia when you have a specific phobia. The absence of research is probably because when the feared thing is not present, your sleep is probably not more disturbed than anyone else's. If you do develop insomnia, CBT-I is likely to work.

Posttraumatic stress

Posttraumatic Stress Disorder (PTSD) is a set of symptoms that occurs following exposure to a terrifying event in which there was a severe threat to personal safety, such as rape, abuse, war, and disasters. Symptoms can include persistent frightening thoughts, memories, and images related to the event, feeling detached and numb, being angry or irritable, and being "jumpy" (easily startled). PTSD can be very disabling. There are various therapeutic approaches and you need to receive help from your family physician and/or a mental health professional in order to get the right treatment for you. With PTSD, sleep is usually very disturbed and you may have frequent nightmares. While the best interventions for posttraumatic nightmares have not yet been clearly identified, some behavioral- and exposure-based techniques seem to be helpful. For example, writing out the nightmare, changing its ending, and rehearsing the new dream ("dream imagery rehearsal") is one of these techniques. The research is limited, but it suggests that CBT-I also improves sleep for people with PTSD. For example, a study from Duke University and the Durham VA Center showed that CBT-I worked for participants with mental health problems, many of whom had combat-related PTSD.

Remember Marie, the woman who became depressed after losing her job? One day, her 18-year-old daughter said, "I think you should see your doctor. I'll drive you if you make the appointment." Marie decided to pick up the phone. That was her first step on her path to feeling better. Over the next few weeks, there were ups and downs, but with medication, help from a psychotherapist, and then with CBT-I, she started to feel like her old self. Last I heard, Marie was preparing her resumé and was feeling hopeful.

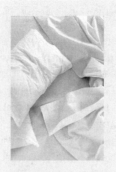

Chapter 22

Sleeping Pills Have a Role:
The Pros and Cons

"Curled in an attitude of peaceful contentment, the princess lies in deep slumber, her head on an ancient, dusty pillow."

George Balanchine

This describes the sleep state of Princess Aurora, the Sleeping Beauty, a sleep that began with a prick of the finger on a spindle supplied by the evil fairy Carabosse. Don't worry, Aurora is soon to be awakened by a prince's kiss. Sleeping potions and spells have figured prominently in fairy tales and other stories for as long as they have been written. Even Harry Potter used a "dreamless sleep potion" to aid his recovery after confronting Voldemort. These stories illustrate our fascination with the medicinal and magical methods of inducing sleep.

It would be nice to think that by simply taking a substance, we could sink into a satisfying and restorative sleep. The truth is, this can happen in some circumstances; in many circumstances a substance is not the best solution. I will go over the advantages and disadvantages of the current medications that are used for sleep to provide you with some basic background information.

As a psychologist, I do not prescribe medication myself. The information that I will review here is based on research and other scientific literature on sleep medications, and I will be covering *general* findings. For your specific situation, you need to consult with your physician and/or pharmacist for personalized advice that will take into account your age, medical history, current medical and psychiatric conditions, other medications, and other factors that are specific to you. Also, the availability of medications depends on the country in which you live. What's available in Canada, where I live, may be different from what's available where you live. I will try to take into account these variations from country to country, but this information is changing all the time. You can get up-to-date information from a pharmacist in your community or, for medications available in the United States, at www.nlm.nih.gov/medlineplus/druginformation.html.

In the sections to follow I will use the term "chronic insomnia" to mean insomnia that has lasted for at least 1 month.

PRESCRIBED SLEEP MEDICATION

The Benzodiazepine Receptor Agonists

These days, if your doctor prescribes a medication to help you sleep, it is most likely to be a benzodiazepine receptor agonist (BzRA). The BzRAs work by promoting the neurotransmitter GABA (gaba-aminobutyric acid), which reduces excitability in the brain. If your brain is in a less excited state, you are more likely to be able to sleep. Here is a table of BzRAs that are commonly prescribed for insomnia. You will see that there are two categories of BzRAs: the "z-drugs" and the "benzodiazepines."

Type of BzRA	Generic Name	Trade Name(s)
z-drug	eszopiclone	Lunesta
z-drug	zopiclone	Imovane
z-drug	zaleplon	Starnoc
z-drug	zolpidem	Ambien, Sublinox, Intermezzo
benzodiazepine	temazepam	Restoril

The z-drugs are named for the z in their names and to distinguish them from the benzodiazepines, an older class of BzRAs. The z-drugs work specifically to help sleep, whereas the benzodiazepines have sleep and anti-anxiety effects. Sometimes people are prescribed benzodiazepines like clonazepam, oxazepam, alprazolam, but the one usually prescribed for sleep is temazepam. It has an onset of action and clearance rate from the blood stream that is suited to sleep, whereas other benzodiazepines are shorter- or longer-acting than this, and are used for purposes other than sleep (like anxiety treatment or sedation when you have a medical procedure).

The pros

These medications can help you get some sleep the very night you take them. If you need sleep, this type of medication will help you immediately. For example, say a family member has died, you are grieving and not sleeping much, but you need to arrange a funeral. This is when your physician may suggest one of the BzRAs. Other types of circumstances when your physician may prescribe this type of medication is when you are not able to sleep because you are going through a stressful time, such as a relationship break up, adjusting to a serious medical diagnosis, or having workplace or family issues. Generally, these medications are effective for sleep when you have sleep difficulty at the time of stressful life events.

The cons

The main disadvantages of BzRAs include their side effects and the risks of tolerance, described below. The side effects of BzRAs vary from medication to medication but the most common ones for the whole group are:

- dizziness

- light-headedness

- drowsiness

- ataxia (trouble walking straight)

- memory problems (amnesia for things that happen in the few hours after taking the medication)

- increased risk of driving accidents

- "hangover effect" (grogginess that sometimes occurs the next morning)

For older people, these problems are especially serious as BzRA-induced dizziness and balance problems can lead to a heightened risk of falls. Because of the possible amnesia, these medications can be especially problematic for anyone with memory problems, such as Alzheimer's disease. The chance of side effects is higher with the longer-acting medications (ones that take more time to clear the bloodstream such as clonazepam, nitrazepam, flurazepam, diazepam, and others), with higher doses, and when the medication is taken in the middle of the night rather than at bedtime.[1] So, side effects are less likely to be troublesome with low doses of shorter-acting medications, taken before bed. It is also important to know that the side effects of BzRAs, described above, are made much worse by alcohol; serious adverse events can occur if you combine the two.

After about 2 to 4 weeks of nightly use, some BzRAs may become less effective due to "tolerance." This means the dose you have been taking starts to have less effect, therefore, you need a higher dose to get the same effect. Tolerance is believed to be a general problem with most BzRAs, although some studies of z-drugs like eszopiclone show that effectiveness may be maintained, even after 6 months of use. Until more research makes it clear, most physicians assume that it is unwise to prescribe any of these medications for longer than 2 to 4 weeks. If your doctor prescribes the medication to be taken intermittently (e.g., 0–4 times per week), there may be fewer problems with tolerance. "Rebound insomnia" is sleep

---

[1] This does not apply to medications that are designed to be taken during nighttime awakenings rather than at bedtime, such as zaleplon and a special formulation of zolpidem called Intermezzo.

difficulty that can occur if you have been taking a BzRA every night for more than 4 weeks and then you suddenly stop taking it. Your body has been accustomed to sleeping with the medication, and without it, insomnia bounces back. Not only does your insomnia return but it's worse than your original sleep difficulty. This rebound insomnia can be so unpleasant that people will resume taking the medication for some relief, which just prolongs the "need" for the medication. Sometimes people think this rebound insomnia is proof that they can't sleep on their own without sleep medication. This is untrue; rebound insomnia is a temporary withdrawal effect and it says nothing about your ability to sleep without medication. Some other withdrawal effects that people can encounter, especially with the benzodiazepines, are a temporary increase in anxiety, distress, restlessness, agitation, irritability, and sensitivity to sounds and other sensory information.

A slow taper off the BzRA can prevent rebound insomnia and other withdrawal effects. If you have been using the medication every night for more than 2 weeks, ask your physician or pharmacist for advice on how to reduce the dose in a step-by-step way to avoid withdrawal effects. If you have been taking these medications for months or years, it is very important to do so. At our health team, the pharmacist meets with people who are wishing to reduce or discontinue BzRA use. He provides useful information about the process and designs schedules to help people slowly taper off the medication. Depending on the usual dose of the medication taken, it can sometimes take several weeks or months until the person is not taking the medication anymore. This type of tapering works best when you have strategies for sleeping without medication, and this is where Sleep Therapy (CBT-I) comes in. With Sleep Therapy you will know what to do if you have a bad night and you will learn how to sleep without the need for medication.

The Sedating Antidepressants

Sometimes, instead of prescribing a BzRA for sleep, physicians prescribe a low dose of an antidepressant medication that has sedative properties. The typical ones are shown here.

Generic name	Trade name(s)
trazodone	Deseryl and various others
doxepin	Sinequan and various others
amitriptyline	Elavil and various others
mirtazapine	Remeron and various others

The pros

These medications do not have the same issues with tolerance as the BzRAs; therefore, they can be taken for longer periods of time at the same dose without losing effectiveness. They may be helpful if you have both depression and insomnia.

The cons

These medications are designed to treat depression, so research on their effectiveness has focused mainly on depressed people. There are almost no studies of whether these medications work at various dosages to treat insomnia in people who are *not* depressed. There are likewise almost no studies of the safety of these medications as used to treat insomnia. Side effects that can occur at the higher doses prescribed for depression include (depending on the specific medication):

- drowsiness

- dizziness

- confusion

- blurred vision

- dry mouth

- constipation

- urinary retention (inability to empty the bladder)

- weight gain

- orthostatic hypotension (low blood pressure when you stand up)

- heart rhythm problems.

In general, sleep specialists believe these medications are more risky than the BzRAs for people with insomnia.

MEDICATIONS PRESCRIBED FOR SLEEP IN SOME COUNTRIES

Melatonin-Based Products

Melatonin is a hormone that is released from the tiny pineal gland in our brain when we are in darkness. It is involved in the regulation of the timing of our sleep. A synthetic melatonin called "exogenous" (outside the body) melatonin is manufactured, which mimics the natural "endogenous" (inside the body) hormone. Ramelteon is what's called a "melatonin-receptor agonist." This means that it promotes melatonin's actions in the brain.

Type	Name
Exogenous melatonin	melatonin
Exogenous melatonin that is released from the capsule over time, rather than all at once	prolonged-release melatonin
Melatonin-receptor agonist	ramelteon

The pros

Prolonged-release melatonin seems to be helpful for insomnia in some people. It has been studied most in older people and is prescribed in Europe for people who are 55 or older. Ramelteon may be helpful for some people who have chronic trouble falling asleep at the beginning of the night. Possible side effects of this group of medications (headache, dizziness, nausea, drowsiness) are usually not a problem; certainly they are less obvious than side effects of BzRAs and antidepressants.

The cons

Standard (immediate-release) melatonin can sometimes be useful for prevention of east-bound jet lag and for certain shift work schedules, and it may be helpful in the short term (1–2 weeks) for insomnia, but it is generally not useful for chronic insomnia. Although prolonged-release melatonin and ramelteon show some promise for insomnia, they have not been studied thoroughly for long-term effects in different age groups, and they are not available in many countries. As a group, these medications appear to be safe in the short term but are lacking long-term safety data. Because they mimic a natural hormone, we do not know how they may affect other biological systems like reproductive hormones, immune functions and circadian rhythms.

NON PRESCRIBED SLEEP MEDICATIONS

Over-the-Counter Sleep Aids

When I first see people in the clinic, I ask what they have used in the past to treat their insomnia. Many people have tried over-the-counter sleep aids. Here is a list of some common ones.

Type	Name of active drug	Trade name(s)
antihistamine	diphenhydramine	Nytol Benadryl Tylenol PM Excedrin PM Advil PM Unisom gel caps and others
antihistamine	doxylamine	Unisom tablets Wal Som
antihistamine	dimenhydrinate	Dramamine Gravol and others

The pros

These medications are available in many drugstores and no prescription is needed. If you have seasonal allergies, these medications may help your sleep on those nights when your allergy symptoms would otherwise disturb your sleep.

The cons

Most of these sleep remedies rely on the drowsiness-inducing effects of sedating antihistamines. They might help you doze off and might even help you to sleep overnight for a few days, but there is little evidence that they are useful for chronic insomnia. Antihistamines are normally used to treat allergic symptoms like runny nose, nasal congestion, and itchiness. If taken for sleep, they will exert their anti histamine effects in the body even when you don't need these effects. Side effects include:

- dry mouth
- increased heart rate
- constipation
- urinary retention
- reduced attention and concentration
- coordination problems
- daytime sedation

Dimenhydrinate (Dramamine or Gravol) is normally used to prevent nausea. Although it can cause drowsiness, we don't know much about its effects on sleep. It has similar side effects to those listed above, and is not recommended for chronic insomnia. All these antihistamine-based medications are especially risky for older people who are more apt to experience mental "fogginess" and balance problems, especially if they already are prone to such symptoms.

Natural Health Products

Here is a table of some natural health products that are sometimes used for sleep.

Type	Name
herbal	valerian
herbal	hops
herbal	kava kava
herbal	lavender
amino acid (building block of protein)	L-tryptophan

The pros

These preparations can be obtained fairly easily at health product stores (apart from high doses or non-oral administration of L-tryptophan, which need a prescription). L-tryptophan does *not* appear to have troublesome side effects, morning "hangover," or tolerance. It may help induce sleepiness and help some people who have mild difficulty falling asleep, and who are otherwise healthy (i.e., no medical or mental health problems).

The cons

At this time there is insufficient evidence of effectiveness for most herbal products for insomnia, mainly because they haven't been well studied. A published review of research on valerian concluded that it is relatively safe, but not effective for insomnia. Use caution when trying herbal products because they are not regulated in the same way that prescription medications are, and information about effectiveness, optimal doses, and adverse effects from stringent clinical trials is often not available. The term "natural" product does not mean the same thing as safe. Some can have dangerous side effects, for example, kava kava can cause liver toxicity.

There are very few recent, rigorous studies of L-tryptophan, so it is difficult to make conclusions about its usefulness for insomnia. Several studies were done in the 1980s and their results were mixed—sometimes L-tryptophan was better than placebo (non active comparison pill), and sometimes it wasn't. In general, there is not much clear evidence that L-tryptophan is useful for chronic insomnia.

ALL TOGETHER

Unlike Sleeping Beauty's sleep in which she stirs, wakens, and falls in love with the Prince, most real-life sleep substances come with side effects. Effects like morning "hangover" are common with the BzRAs and the sedating antidepressants. Melatonin-based products and L-tryptophan seem to have fewer side effects but their effectiveness is not well established, especially for L-tryptophan. There is no convincing evidence for herbal sleep remedies. Although some medications are helpful in the short term (e.g., the BzRAs), no sleeping medication has shown itself to be entirely useful for chronic insomnia. Also, the timing and amount of certain sleep stages (see Appendix A) such as REM sleep can be affected by medications, especially the BzRAs and the antidepressants. This means that the sleep you get with the medication is somewhat different from what your sleep would be if you were sleeping well without medication. If sleep medication *does* work, its effects don't last after the medication is discontinued; it does not cure insomnia. Sleep medication is not a long-term answer for persistent insomnia.

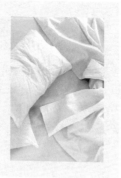

Afterword

Good Luck and Good Night

Several people have joked since this project began, "I hope your book puts people to sleep!" Usually falling asleep in response to someone's writing is not a good sign. But in this case, I'll take it as a sign that this book has done its job. So I sincerely hope it *has* put you to sleep, by showing you how to solve your insomnia. Good luck, and remember: no chasing after sleep. All that is required is to make the circumstances conducive to sleep by using the tried-and-true techniques found here, and then relax, occupy your mind with other things, and be delighted when sleep arrives. Good luck and best wishes for a good night.

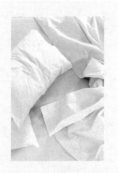

Bibliography

PREFACE

Davidson, J. R., Aimé, A., Ivers, H., & Morin, C. M. (2009). Characteristics of individuals with insomnia who seek treatment in a clinical setting versus those who volunteer for a randomized controlled trial. *Behavioral Sleep Medicine, 7,* 37-52.

Davidson, J. R., MacLean, A. W., Brundage, M. D., & Schultze, K. (2002). Sleep disturbance in cancer patients. *Social Science and Medicine, 54,* 1309-1321.

Davidson, J. R., Waisberg, J. L., Brundage, M. D., & MacLean, A. W. (2001). Nonpharmacologic group treatment of insomnia: A preliminary study with cancer survivors. *Psycho-Oncology, 10,* 389-397.

Moldofsky, H., Lue, F. A., Davidson, J. R., & Gorczynski, R. (1989). Effects of sleep deprivation on human immune functions. *Federation of American Societies for Experimental Biology (FASEB) Journal, 3,* 1972-1977.

CHAPTER 1

Davidson, J. R., Aimé, A., Ivers, H., & Morin, C. M. (2009). Characteristics of individuals with insomnia who seek treatment in a clinical setting versus those who volunteer for a randomized controlled trial. *Behavioral Sleep Medicine, 7,* 37-52.

Espie, C. A., Inglis, S. J., Tessier, S., & Harvey, L. (2001). The clinical effectiveness of cognitive behaviour therapy for chronic insomnia: Implementation and evaluation of a sleep clinic in general medical practice. *Behaviour Research and Therapy, 39,* 45-60.

Lichstein, K. L., Stone, K. C., Nau, S. D., McCrae, C. S., & Payne, K. L. (2006). Insomnia in the elderly. *Sleep Medicine Clinics, 1,* 221-229.

Montagna, P., & Provini, F. (2008). Prion disorders and sleep. *Sleep Medicine Clinics, 3*, 411–426.

Morgenthaler, T., Kramer, M., Alessi, C., Friedman, L., Boehlecke, B., Brown, T., Coleman, J., Kapur, V., Lee-Chong, T., Owens, J., Pancer, J., Swick, T., & American Academy of Sleep Medicine (2006). Practice parameters for the psychological and behavioral treatment of insomnia: An update. An American Academy of Sleep Medicine Report. *Sleep, 29*, 1415–1419.

Morin, C. M., & Benca, R. (2012). Chronic insomnia. *The Lancet, 379*, 1129–1141.

Morin, C. M., Colecchi, C., Stone, J., Sood, R., & Brink, D. (1999). Behavioral and pharmacological therapies for late-life insomnia: A randomized controlled trial. *Journal of the American Medical Association, 281*, 991–999.

Morin, C. M., Culbert, J. P., & Schwartz, S. M. (1994). Nonpharmacological interventions for insomnia: A meta-analysis of treatment efficacy. *The American Journal of Psychiatry, 151*, 1172–1180.

Murtagh, D. R., & Greenwood, K. M. (1995). Identifying effective psychological treatments for insomnia: A meta-analysis. *Journal of Consulting and Clinical Psychology, 63*, 79–89.

National Institutes of Health (2005). State of the Science Conference Statement on manifestations and management of chronic insomnia in adults, June 13–15, 2005. *Sleep, 28*, 1049–1057.

Rybarczyk, B., Stepanski, E., Fogg, L., Lopez, M., Barry, P., & Davis, A. (2005). A placebo-controlled test of cognitive-behavioral therapy for comorbid insomnia in older adults. *Journal of Consulting and Clinical Psychology, 73*, 1164–1174.

Schutte-Rodin, S., Broch, L., Buysse, D., Dorsey, C., & Sateia, M. (2008). Clinical guideline for the evaluation and management of chronic insomnia in adults. *Journal of Clinical Sleep Medicine, 4*, 487–504.

Smith, M. T., Huang, M. I., & Manber, R. (2005). Cognitive behavior therapy for chronic insomnia occurring within the context of medical and psychiatric disorders. *Clinical Psychology Review, 25*, 559–592.

Wilson, S. J., Nutt, D. J., Alford, C., Argyropoulos, S. V., Baldwin, D. S., Bateson, A. N., Britton, T. C., Crowe, C., Dijk, D.-J., Espie, C. A., Gringras, P., Hajak, G., Idzikowski, C., Krystal, A. D., Nash, J. R., Selsick, H., Sharpley, A. L., & Wade, A. G. (2010). British Association for Psychopharmacology consensus statement on evidence-based treatment of insomnia, parasomnias and circadian rhythm disorders. *Journal of Psychopharmacology, 24*, 1577–1600.

CHAPTER 2

American Academy of Sleep Medicine. (2005). *International classification of sleep disorders: Diagnostic and coding manual* (2nd ed.). Westchester: American Academy of Sleep Medicine.

American Psychiatric Association. DSM-5 Development. (2012). Sleep-wake disorders, insomnia disorder, proposed revision and rationale. Retrieved May 1, 2012 from http://www.dsm5.org/ProposedRevision/Pages/proposedrevision.aspx?rid=65

Anderson, J. R. (2000). Sleep-related behavioural adaptations in free-ranging anthropoid primates. *Sleep Medicine Reviews, 4*, 355–373.

Morin, C. M., LeBlanc, M., Daley, M., Gregoire, J. P., & Mérette, C. (2006). Epidemiology of insomnia: Prevalence, self-help treatments, consultations, and determinants of help-seeking behaviors. *Sleep Medicine, 7,* 123-130.

Riedel, B. W., & Lichstein, K. L. (2000). Insomnia and daytime functioning. *Sleep Medicine Reviews, 4,* 277-298.

Shekleton, J. A., Rogers, N. L., & Rajaratnam, S. M. W. (2010). Searching for the daytime impairments of primary insomnia. *Sleep Medicine Reviews, 14,* 47-60.

Walsh, J. K. (2004). Clinical and socioeconomic correlates of insomnia. *Journal of Clinical Psychiatry, 65*(Suppl. 8), 13-19.

Zammit, G. K., Weiner, J., Damato, N., Sillup, G. P., & McMillan, C. A. (1999). Quality of life in people with insomnia. *Sleep, 22,* S379-S385.

CHAPTER 3

Basner, M. (2010). Is time for sleep declining among Americans? *Sleep, 33,* 13-14.

Basner, M., & Dinges, D. F. (2009). Dubious bargain: Trading sleep for Leno and Letterman. *Sleep, 32,* 747-752.

Brody, J. E. (1994, January 19). Personal health: Health alarm for a sleep-deprived society. *The New York Times.*

Bryant, P. A., Trinder, J., & Curtis, N. (2004). Sick and tired: Does sleep have a vital role in the immune system? *Nature Reviews Immunology, 4,* 457-467.

Ekirch, A. R. (2001). Sleep we have lost: Pre-industrial slumber in the British Isles. *American Historical Review, 106,* 343-386.

Groeger, J. A., Zijlstra, F. R. H., & Dijk, D.-J. (2004). Sleep quantity, sleep difficulties and their perceived consequences in a representative sample of some 2000 British adults. *Journal of Sleep Research, 13,* 359-371.

Irwin, M. (2002). Effects of sleep and sleep loss on immunity and cytokines. *Brain, Behavior, and Immunity, 16,* 503-512.

Jean-Louis, G., Kripke, D. F., Ancoli-Israel, S., Klauber, M. R., & Sepulveda, R. S. (2000). Sleep duration, illumination, and activity patterns in a population sample: Effects of gender and ethnicity. *Biological Psychiatry, 47,* 921-927.

Knutson, K. L., Van Cauter, E., Rathouz, P. J., DeLeire, T., & Lauderdale, D. S. (2010). Trends in the prevalence of short sleepers in the USA: 1975-2006. *Sleep, 33,* 37-45.

Kronholm, E., Partonen, T., Laatikainen, T., Peltonen, M., Härmä, M., Hublin, C., Kaprio, J., Aro, A. R., Partinen, M., Fogelholm, M., Valve, R., Vahtera, J., Oksanen, T., Kivimäki, M., Koskenvuo, M., & Sutela, H. (2008). Trends in self-reported sleep duration and insomnia-related symptoms in Finland from 1972 to 2005: A comparative review and re-analysis of Finnish population samples. *Journal of Sleep Research, 17,* 54-62.

Krueger, P. M., & Friedman, E. M. (2009). Sleep duration in the United States: A cross-sectional population-based study. *American Journal of Epidemiology, 169,* 1052-1063.

Luckhaupt, S. E., Tak, S., & Calvert, G. M. (2010). The prevalence of short sleep duration by industry and occupation in the National Health Interview Survey. *Sleep, 33,* 149-159.

Meerlo, P., Sgoifo, A., & Suchecki, D. (2008). Restricted and disrupted sleep: Effects on autonomic function, neuroendocrine stress systems and stress responsivity. *Sleep Medicine Reviews, 12,* 197-210.

Orff, H. J., Drummond, S. P. A., Nowakowski, S., & Perlis, M. L. (2007). Discrepancy between subjective symptomatology and objective neuropsychological performance in insomnia. *Sleep, 30*, 1205-1211.

Semler, C. N., & Harvey, A. G. (2006). Daytime functioning in primary insomnia: Does attentional focus contribute to *real* or *perceived* impairment? *Behavioral Sleep Medicine, 4*, 85-103.

Van Dongen, H. P. A., Maislin, G., Mullington, J. M., & Dinges, D. F. (2003). The cumulative cost of additional wakefulness: Dose-response effects on neurobehavioral functions and sleep physiology from chronic sleep restriction and total sleep deprivation. *Sleep, 26*, 117-126.

Varkevisser, M., Van Dongen, H. P. A., Van Amsterdam, J. G. C., & Kerkhof, G. A. (2007). Chronic insomnia and daytime functioning: An ambulatory assessment. *Behavioral Sleep Medicine, 5*, 279-296.

Virtanen, M., Ferrie, J. E., Gimeno, D., Vahtera, J., Elovainio, M., Singh-Manoux, A., Marmot, M. G., & Kivimäki, M. (2009). Long working hours and sleep disturbances: The Whitehall II Prospective Cohort Study. *Sleep, 32*, 737-745.

CHAPTER 9

Aber, R., & Webb, W. B. (1986). Effects of a limited nap on night sleep in older subjects. *Psychology of Aging, 1*, 300-302.

Aschoff, J. (1994). Naps as integral parts of the wake time within the human sleep-wake cycle. *Journal of Biological Rhythms, 9*, 145-155.

Dinges, D. F., & Broughton, R. J. (Eds.). (1989). *Sleep and alertness: Chronobiological, behavioral, and medical aspects of napping.* New York, NY: Raven Press.

Gordis, E. (1997). *Alcohol metabolism* (Alcohol Alert No. 35). Retrieved June 3, 2012, from http://pubs.niaaa.nih.gov/publications/aa35.htm

Landolt, H.-P., Roth, C., Dijk, D.-J., & Borbély, A. A. (1996). Late-afternoon ethanol intake affects nocturnal sleep and the sleep EEG in middle-aged men. *Journal of Clinical Psychopharmacology, 16*, 428-436.

Madsen, B. W., & Rossi, L. (1980). Sleep and Michaelis-Menten elimination of ethanol. *Clinical Pharmacology & Therapeutics, 27*, 114-119.

National Institute on Alcohol Abuse and Alcoholism. (1998). *Alcohol and sleep* (Alcohol Alert No. 41). Retrieved December 17, 2011, from http://pubs.niaaa.nih.gov/publications/aa41.htm

Ramchandani, V. A., Bosron, W. F., & Li, T. K. (2001). Research advances in ethanol metabolism. *Pathologie Biologie (Paris), 49*, 676-682.

Roehrs, T., & Roth, T. (2011). *Sleep, sleepiness, and alcohol use.* Retrieved June 3, 2012, from http://pubs.niaaa.nih.gov/publications/arh25-2/101-109.htm

Taberner, P. V. (1988). Pharmacokinetics of alcohol and the law. *Trends in Pharmacological Sciences, 9*, 47-48.

Wilkinson, P. K., Sedman, A. J., Sakmar, E., Kay, D. R., & Wagner, J. G. (1977). Pharmacokinetics of ethanol after oral administration in the fasting state. *Journal of Pharmacokinetics and Biopharmaceutics, 5*, 207-224.

CHAPTER 10

Bootzin, R. R. (1972). Stimulus control treatment for insomnia. *Proceedings of the American Psychological Association, 7*, 395-396.

Borbély, A. A. (1982). A two process model of sleep regulation. *Human Neurobiology, 1*, 195-204.

Spielman, A. J., Saskin, P., & Thorpy, M. J. (1987). Treatment of chronic insomnia by restriction of time in bed. *Sleep, 10*, 45-56.

CHAPTER 16

Rowley, J. T., Stickgold, R., & Hobson, J. A. (1998). Eyelid movements and mental activity at sleep onset. *Consciousness and Cognition, 7*, 67-84.

Stickgold, R., Malia, A., Maguire, D., Roddenberry, D., & O'Connor, M. (2000). Replaying the game: Hypnagogic images in normals and amnesics. *Science, 290*, 350-353.

CHAPTER 17

Morin, C. M., Colecchi, C., Stone, J., Sood, R., & Brink, D. (1999). Behavioral and pharmacological therapies for late-life insomnia: A randomized controlled trial. *Journal of the American Medical Association, 281*, 991-999.

CHAPTER 18

Ancoli-Israel, S., Kripke, D. F., Klauber, M. R., Mason, W. J., Fell, R., & Kaplan, O. (1991). Periodic limb movements in sleep in community-dwelling elderly. *Sleep, 14*, 496-500.

Ancoli-Israel, S., Kripke, D. F., Klauber, M. R., Mason, W. J., Fell, R., & Kaplan, O. (1991). Sleep-disordered breathing in community-dwelling elderly. *Sleep, 14*, 486-495.

Baker, F. C., Lamarche, L. J., Iacovides, S., & Colrain, I. M. (2008). Sleep and menstrual-related disorders. In H. S. Driver (Ed.), *Sleep and disorders of sleep in women* (pp. 25-35). Philadelphia, PA: Elsevier.

Bliwise, D. L. (2009). Restless legs syndrome and periodic limb movements in the elderly with and without dementia. In W. A. Hening, R. P. Allen, S. Chokroverty, & C. J. Earley (Eds.), *Restless legs syndrome* (pp. 178-184). Philadelphia, PA: Saunders.

Boergers, J., Hart, C., Owens, J. A., Streisand, R., & Spirito, A. (2007). Child sleep disorders: Associations with parental sleep duration and daytime sleepiness. *Journal of Family Psychology, 21*, 88-94.

Cartwright, R., & Lamberg, L. (1992). *Crisis dreaming: Using your dreams to solve your problems*. New York, NY: HarperCollins.

Crowley, K. (2011). Sleep and sleep disorders in older adults. *Neuropsychology Review, 21*, 41-53.

Davidson, J. R. (2008). Insomnia: Therapeutic options for women. In H. S. Driver (Ed.), *Sleep and disorders of sleep in women* (pp. 109-119). Philadelphia, PA: Elsevier.

Driver, H. S., Werth, E., Dijk, D.-J., & Borbély, A. A. (2008). The menstrual cycle effects on sleep. In H. S. Driver (Ed.), *Sleep and disorders of sleep in women* (pp. 1–11). Philadelphia, PA: Elsevier.

Edwards, N., & Sullivan, C. E. (2008). Sleep-disordered breathing in pregnancy. In H. S. Driver (Ed.), *Sleep and disorders of sleep in women* (pp. 81–95). Philadelphia, PA: Elsevier.

Greenberg, J. (2006). Losing sleep over organizational injustice: Attenuating insomniac reactions to underpayment inequity with supervisory training in interactional justice. *Journal of Applied Psychology, 91*, 58–69.

Hall, W. A., Hauck, Y. L., Carty, E. M., Hutton, E. K., Fenwick, J., & Stoll, K. (2009). Childbirth fear, anxiety, fatigue, and sleep deprivation in pregnant women. *Journal of Obstetric, Gynecologic, & Neonatal Nursing, 38*, 567–576.

Harvard Medical School. (2010). *Medications that can affect sleep.* Retrieved November 16, 2011, from http://www.health.harvard.edu/newsletters/Harvard_Womens_Health_Watch/2010/July/medications-that-can-affect-sleep

Health Canada. (2004). *Benefits and risks of hormone replacement therapy (estrogen with or without progestin).* Retrieved November 16, 2011, from http://www.hc-sc.gc.ca/hl-vs/lyh-vsv/med/estrogen-eng.php

Jansson, M., & Linton, S. J. (2006). Psychosocial work stressors in the development and maintenance of insomnia: A prospective study. *Journal of Occupational Health Psychology, 11*, 241–248.

Jean-Louis, G., Kripke, D. F., Assmus, J. D., & Langer, R. D. (2000). Sleep-wake patterns among postmenopausal women: A 24-hour unattended polysomnographic study. *Journal of Gerontology: Medical Sciences, 55A*, M120–M123.

Johnson, E. O., Roth, T., Schultz, L., & Breslau, N. (2006). Epidemiology of DSM-IV insomnia in adolescence: Lifetime prevalence, chronicity, and an emergent gender difference. *Pediatrics, 117*, e247–e256.

Kloss, J. D., Tweedy, K., & Gilrain, K. (2004). Psychological factors associated with sleep disturbance among perimenopausal women. *Behavioral Sleep Medicine, 2*, 177–190.

Lallukka, T., Rahkonen, O., Lahelma, E., & Arber, S. (2010). Sleep complaints in middle-aged women and men: The contribution of working conditions and work-family conflicts. *Journal of Sleep Research, 19*, 466–477.

Manconi, M., & Ferini-Strambi, L. (2009). Restless legs syndrome and pregnancy. In W. A. Hening, R. P. Allen, S. Chokroverty, & C. J. Earley (Eds.), *Restless legs syndrome* (pp. 173–177). Philadelphia, PA: Saunders.

Meijer, A. M., & Van den Wittenboer, G. L. H. (2007). Contribution of infants' sleep and crying to marital relationship of first-time parent couples in the 1st year after childbirth. *Journal of Family Psychology, 21*, 49–57.

Meltzer, L. J., & Mindell, J. A. (2007). Relationship between child sleep disturbances and maternal sleep, mood, and parenting stress: A pilot study. *Journal of Family Psychology, 21*, 67–73.

Mindell, J. A., & Jacobson, B. J. (2000). Sleep disturbances during pregnancy. *Journal of Obstetric, Gynecologic, & Neonatal Nursing, 29*, 590–597.

Moline, M. L., Broch, L., Zak, R., & Gross, V. (2003). Sleep in women across the life cycle from adulthood through menopause. *Sleep Medicine Reviews, 7*, 155–177.

Nielsen, T., & Paquette, T. (2007). Dream-associated behaviors affecting pregnant and postpartum women. *Sleep, 30,* 1162–1169.

Ohayon, M. M., Roberts, R. E., Zulley, J., Smirne, S., & Priest, R. G. (2000). Prevalence and patterns of problematic sleep among older adolescents. *Journal of the American Academy of Child & Adolescent Psychiatry, 39,* 1549–1556.

Polo-Kantola, P. (2008). Dealing with menopausal sleep disturbances. In H. S. Driver (Ed.), *Sleep and disorders of sleep in women* (pp. 121–131). Philadelphia, PA: Elsevier.

Provini, F., Vetrugno, R., Ferri, R., & Montagna, P. (2009). Periodic limb movements in sleep. In W. A. Hening, R. P. Allen, S. Chokroverty, & C. J. Earley (Eds.), *Restless legs syndrome* (pp. 119–133). Philadelphia, PA: Saunders.

Santiago, J. R., Nolledo, M. S., Kinzler, W., & Santiago, T. V. (2001). Sleep and sleep disorders in pregnancy. *Annals of Internal Medicine, 134,* 396–408.

Savard, J., Davidson, J. R., Ivers, H., Quesnel, C., Rioux, D., Dupéré, V., Lasnier, M., Simard, S., & Morin, C. M. (2004). The association between nocturnal hot flashes and sleep in breast cancer survivors. *Journal of Pain and Symptom Management, 27,* 513–522.

Savard, J., Simard, S., Ivers, H., & Morin, C. M. (2005). Randomized study on the efficacy of cognitive-behavioral therapy for insomnia secondary to breast cancer, part I: Sleep and psychological effects. *Journal of Clinical Oncology, 23,* 6083–6096.

Shaver, J. L. F., Johnston, S. K., Lentz, M. J., & Landis, C. A. (2002). Stress exposure, psychological distress, and physiological stress activation in midlife women with insomnia. *Psychosomatic Medicine, 64,* 793–802.

Signal, T. L., Gander, P. H., Sangalli, M. R., Travier, N., Firestone, R. T., & Tuohy, J. F. (2007). Sleep duration and quality in healthy nulliparous and multiparous women across pregnancy and post-partum. *Australian and New Zealand Journal of Obstetrics and Gynaecology, 47,* 16–22.

Sloan, E. P. (2008). Sleep disruption during pregnancy. In H. S. Driver (Ed.), *Sleep and disorders of sleep in women* (pp. 73–80). Philadelphia, PA: Elsevier.

Smith, M. T., Perlis, M. L., Park, A., Smith, M. S., Pennington, J., Giles, D. E., & Buysse, D. J. (2002). Comparative meta-analysis of pharmacotherapy and behavior therapy for persistent insomnia. *The American Journal of Psychiatry, 159,* 5–11.

Vitiello, M. V., Larsen, L. H., & Moe, K. E. (2004). Age-related sleep change: Gender and estrogen effects on the subjective-objective sleep quality relationships of healthy, noncomplaining older men and women. *Journal of Psychosomatic Research, 56,* 503–510.

Westerlund, H., Alexanderson, K., Åkerstedt, T., Hanson, L. M., Theorell, T., & Kivimäki, M. (2008). Work-related sleep disturbances and sickness absence in the Swedish working population, 1993–1999. *Sleep, 31,* 1169–1177.

Yoshioka, E., Saijo, Y., Kita, T., Satoh, H., Kawaharada, M., Fukui, T., & Kishi, R. (2012). Gender differences in insomnia and the role of paid work and family responsibilities. *Social Psychiatry and Psychiatric Epidemiology, 47,* 651-662.

Young, T., Finn, L., Austin, D., & Peterson, A. (2003). Menopausal status and sleep-disordered breathing in the Wisconsin Sleep Cohort Study. *American Journal of Respiratory and Critical Care Medicine, 167,* 1181–1185.

CHAPTER 19

Andersen, M. L., & Tufik, S. (2008). The effects of testosterone on sleep and sleep-disordered breathing in men: Its bidirectional interaction with erectile function. *Sleep Medicine Reviews, 12*, 365-379.

Aserinsky, E., & Kleitman, N. (1953). Regularly occurring periods of eye motility, and concomitant phenomena, during sleep. *Science, 118*, 273-274.

Bixler, E. O., Papaliaga, M. N., Vgontzas, A. N., Lin, H.-M., Pejovic, S., Karataraki, M., Vela-Bueno, A., & Chrousos, G. P. (2009). Women sleep objectively better than men and the sleep of young women is more resilient to external stressors: Effects of age and menopause. *Journal of Sleep Research, 18*, 221-228.

Brissette, S., Montplaisir, J., Godbout, R., & Lavoisier, P. (1985). Sexual activity and sleep in humans. *Biological Psychiatry, 20*, 758-763.

Driver, H. S. (2012). Sleep and gender: The paradox of sex and sleep? In C. M. Morin & C. A. Espie (Eds.), *The Oxford handbook of sleep and sleep disorders* (pp. 266-288). New York, NY: Oxford University Press.

Driver, H. S., & Taylor, S. R. (2000). Exercise and sleep. *Sleep Medicine Reviews, 4*, 387-402.

Elliott, S., Latini, D. M., Walker, L. M., Wassersug, R., Robinson, J. W., & The ADT Survivorship Working Group. (2010). Androgen deprivation therapy for prostate cancer: Recommendations to improve patient and partner quality of life. *The Journal of Sexual Medicine, 7*, 2996-3010.

Gordon, S. (2012, May 5). On thin ice. *The Globe and Mail*.

Handelsman, D. J., & Liu, P. Y. (2005). Andropause: Invention, prevention, rejuvenation. *Trends in Endocrinology and Metabolism, 16*, 39-45.

Heaton, J. P. W. (2003). Hormone treatments and preventative strategies in the aging male: Whom and when to treat? *Reviews in Urology, 5*, S16-S21.

Hoffstein, V. (2005). Snoring and upper airway resistance. In M. H. Kryger, T. Roth, & W. C. Dement (Eds.), *Principles and practice of sleep medicine* (4th ed., pp. 1001-1012). Philadelphia, PA: Elsevier Saunders.

Janson, C., Lindberg, E., Gislason, T., Elmasry, A., & Boman, G. (2001). Insomnia in men: A 10-year prospective population based study. *Sleep, 24*, 425-430.

Kruger, D. J., & Hughes, S. M. (2011). Tendencies to fall asleep first after sex are associated with greater partner desires for bonding and affection. *Journal of Social, Evolutionary, and Cultural Psychology, 5*, 239-247.

Mills, J. N., Minors, D. S., & Waterhouse, J. M. (1974). The circadian rhythms of human subjects without timepieces or indication of the alternation of day and night. *Journal of Physiology, 240*, 567-594.

Montgomery, P., & Dennis, J. A. (2009). Physical exercise for sleep problems in adults aged 60+. *The Cochrane Library, 1*, 1-14.

Savard, J., Simard, S., Hervouet, S., Ivers, H., Lacombe, L., & Fradet, Y. (2005). Insomnia in men treated with radical prostatectomy for prostate cancer. *Psycho-Oncology, 14*, 147-156.

Schmidt, M. H. (2005). Neural mechanisms of sleep-related penile erections. In M. H. Kryger, T. Roth, & W. C. Dement (Eds.), *Principles and practice of sleep medicine* (4th ed., pp. 305-317). Philadelphia, PA: Elsevier Saunders.

Siffre, M. (1964). *Beyond time.* (1st ed.). New York, NY: McGraw-Hill.

Strollo, P. J., Atwood, C. W., & Sanders, M. H. (2005). Medical therapy for obstructive sleep apnea-hypopnea syndrome. In M. H. Kryger, T. Roth, & W. C. Dement (Eds.), *Principles and practice of sleep medicine* (4th ed., pp. 1053–1065). Philadelphia, PA: Elsevier Saunders.

Tariq, S. H., Haren, M. T., Kim, M. J., & Morley, J. E. (2005). Andropause: Is the emperor wearing any clothes? *Reviews in Endocrine & Metabolic Disorders, 6,* 77–84.

Vitiello, M. V., Larsen, L. H., & Moe, K. E. (2004). Age-related sleep change: Gender and estrogen effects on the subjective-objective sleep quality relationships of healthy, noncomplaining older men and women. *Journal of Psychosomatic Research, 56,* 503–510.

Walker, L. M., & Robinson, J. W. (2011). A description of heterosexual couples' sexual adjustment to androgen deprivation therapy for prostate cancer. *Psycho-Oncology, 20,* 880–888.

Ware, J.C., & Hirshkowitz, M. (2005) Assessment of sleep-related erections. In M.H. Kryger, T. Roth, & W.C. Dement (Eds.), Principles and practice of sleep medicine (4th ed., pp.1394–1402). Philadelphia, PA: Elsevier Saunders. Webb, W. B., & Agnew, H. W. (1965). Sleep: Effects of a restricted regime. *Science, 150,* 1745–1747.

Young, T., Palta, M., Dempsey, J., Skatrud, J., Weber, S., & Badr, S. (1993). The occurrence of sleep-disordered breathing among middle-aged adults. *The New England Journal of Medicine, 328,* 1230–1235.

Youngstedt, S. D. (2005). Effects of exercise on sleep. *Clinics in Sports Medicine, 24,* 355–365.

Zhang, B., & Wing, Y.-K. (2006). Sex differences in insomnia: A meta-analysis. *Sleep, 29,* 85–93.

CHAPTER 20

General

Davidson, J. R., Aimé, A., Ivers, H., & Morin, C. M. (2009). Characteristics of individuals with insomnia who seek treatment in a clinical setting versus those who volunteer for a randomized controlled trial. *Behavioral Sleep Medicine, 7,* 37–52.

Fleming, L., & Davidson, J. R. (2012). Sleep and medical disorders. In C. M. Morin & C. A. Espie (Eds.), *The Oxford handbook of sleep and sleep disorders* (pp. 502-525). New York, NY: Oxford University Press.

Rybarczyk, B., Stepanski, E., Fogg, L., Lopez, M., Barry, P., & Davis, A. (2005). A placebo-controlled test of cognitive-behavioral therapy for comorbid insomnia in older adults. *Journal of Consulting and Clinical Psychology, 73,* 1164–1174.

Smith, M. T., Huang, M. I., & Manber, R. (2005). Cognitive behavior therapy for chronic insomnia occurring within the context of medical and psychiatric disorders. *Clinical Psychology Review, 25,* 559–592.

Taylor, D. J., Mallory, L. J., Lichstein, K. L., Durrence, H. H., Riedel, B. W., & Bush, A. J. (2007). Comorbidity of chronic insomnia with medical problems. *Sleep, 30,* 213–218.

Walsh, J. K., Coulouvrat, C., Hajak, G., Lakoma, M. D., Petukhova, M., Roth, T., Sampson, N. A., Shahly, V., Shillington, A., Stephenson, J. J., & Kessler, R. C. (2011). Nighttime insomnia symptoms and perceived health in the America Insomnia Survey (AIS). *Sleep, 34,* 997–1011.

Chronic Pain

Currie, S. R., Wilson, K. G., Pontefract, A. J., & deLaplante, L. (2000). Cognitive-behavioral treatment of insomnia secondary to chronic pain. *Journal of Consulting and Clinical Psychology, 68,* 407–416.

Edinger, J. D., Wohlgemuth, W. K., Krystal, A. D., & Rice, J. R. (2005). Behavioral insomnia therapy for fibromyalgia patients: A randomized clinical trial. *Archives of Internal Medicine, 165,* 2527–2535.

Häuser, W., Klose, P., Langhorst, J., Moradi, B., Steinbach, M., Schiltenwolf, M., & Busch, A. (2010). Efficacy of different types of aerobic exercise in fibromyalgia syndrome: A systematic review and meta-analysis of randomised controlled trials. *Arthritis Research & Therapy, 12, Epub R79 - May 10, 2010.*

Menefee, L. A., Cohen, M. J. M., Anderson, W. R., Doghramji, K., Frank, E. D., & Lee, H. (2000). Sleep disturbance and nonmalignant chronic pain: A comprehensive review of the literature. *Pain Medicine, 1,* 156–172.

Rybarczyk, B., Stepanski, E., Fogg, L., Lopez, M., Barry, P., & Davis, A. (2005). A placebo-controlled test of cognitive-behavioral therapy for comorbid insomnia in older adults. *Journal of Consulting and Clinical Psychology, 73,* 1164–1174.

Smith, M. T., & Haythornthwaite, J. A. (2004). How do sleep disturbance and chronic pain inter-relate? Insights from the longitudinal and cognitive-behavioral clinical trials literature. *Sleep Medicine Reviews, 8,* 119–132.

Vitiello, M. V., Rybarczyk, B., Von Korff, M., & Stepanski, E. J. (2009). Cognitive behavioral therapy for insomnia improves sleep and decreases pain in older adults with co-morbid insomnia and osteoarthritis. *Journal of Clinical Sleep Medicine, 5,* 355–362.

Heart Disease

Andreas, S., Schulz, R., Werner, G. S., & Kreuzer, H. (1996). Prevalance of obstructive sleep apnoea in patients with coronary artery disease. *Coronary Artery Disease, 7,* 541–545.

Hedner, J., Franklin, K. A., & Peker, Y. (2007). Obstructive sleep apnea and coronary artery disease. *Sleep Medicine Clinics, 2,* 559–564.

Kaye, J., Kaye, K., & Madow, L. (1983). Sleep patterns in patients with cancer and patients with cardiac disease. *The Journal of Psychology, 114,* 107–113.

Phillips, B. (2005). Sleep-disordered breathing and cardiovascular disease. *Sleep Medicine Reviews, 9,* 131–140.

Rybarczyk, B., Stepanski, E., Fogg, L., Lopez, M., Barry, P., & Davis, A. (2005). A placebo-controlled test of cognitive-behavioral therapy for comorbid insomnia in older adults. *Journal of Consulting and Clinical Psychology, 73,* 1164–1174.

Cancer

Carter, P. A. (2006). A brief behavioral sleep intervention for family caregivers of persons with cancer. *Cancer Nursing, 29,* 95–103.

Davidson, J. R. (2012). Sleep disturbance interventions for oncology patients: Steps forward and issues arising. *Sleep Medicine Reviews, 16,* 395–396.

Davidson, J. R., MacLean, A. W., Brundage, M. D., & Schulze, K. (2002). Sleep disturbance in cancer patients. *Social Science and Medicine, 54*, 1309-1321.

Davidson, J. R., Waisberg, J. L., Brundage, M. D., & MacLean, A. W. (2001). Nonpharmacologic group treatment of insomnia: A preliminary study with cancer survivors. *Psycho-Oncology, 10*, 389-397.

Espie, C. A., Fleming, L., Cassidy, J., Samuel, L., Taylor, L. M., White, C. A., Douglas, N. J., Engleman, H. M., Kelly, H.-L., & Paul, J. (2008). Randomized controlled clinical effectiveness trial of cognitive behavior therapy compared with treatment as usual for persistent insomnia in patients with cancer. *Journal of Clinical Oncology, 26*, 4651-4658.

Langford, D. J., Lee, K., & Miaskowski, C. (2012). Sleep disturbance interventions in oncology patients and family caregivers: A comprehensive review and meta-analysis. *Sleep Medicine Reviews, 16*, 397-414.

Quesnel, C., Savard, J., Simard, S., Ivers, H., & Morin, C. M. (2003). Efficacy of cognitive-behavioral therapy for insomnia in women treated for nonmetastatic breast cancer. *Journal of Consulting and Clinical Psychology, 71*, 189-200.

Savard, J., Simard, S., Ivers, H., & Morin, C. M. (2005). Randomized study on the efficacy of cognitive-behavioral therapy for insomnia secondary to breast cancer, part I: Sleep and psychological effects. *Journal of Clinical Oncology, 23*, 6083-6096.

Seasonal Allergies

Lunn, M., & Craig, T. (2011). Rhinitis and sleep. *Sleep Medicine Reviews, 15*, 293-299.

Meltzer, E. O., Nathan, R., Derebery, J., Stang, P. E., Campbell, U. B., Yeh, W.-S., Corrao, M., Stanford R. Sleep, quality of life, and productivity impact of nasal symptoms in the United States: Findings from the Burden of Rhinitis in *America survey. Allergy and Asthma Proceedings, 30*, 244-254.

Breathing Problems

Budhiraja, R., Parthasarathy, S., Budhiraja, P., Habib, M. P., Wendel, C., & Quan, S. F. (2012). Insomnia in patients with COPD. *Sleep, 35*, 369-375.

Cormick, W., Olson, L. G., Hensley, M. J., & Saunders, N. A. (1986). Nocturnal hypoxaemia and quality of sleep in patients with chronic obstructive lung disease. *Thorax, 41*, 846-854.

Douglas, N. J. (1992). Nocturnal hypoxemia in patients with chronic obstructive pulmonary disease. *Clinics in Chest Medicine, 13*, 523-532.

Fleetham, J., West, P., Mezon, B., Conway, W., Roth, T., & Kryger, M. (1982). Sleep, arousals, and oxygen desaturation in chronic obstructive pulmonary disease: The effect of oxygen therapy. *The American Review of Respiratory Disease, 126*, 429-433.

Kapella, M. C., Herdegen, J. J., Perlis, M. L., Shaver, J. L., Larson, J. L., Law, J. A., & Carley, D. W. (2011). Cognitive behavioral therapy for insomnia comorbid with COPD is feasible with preliminary evidence of positive sleep and fatigue effects. *International Journal of COPD, 6*, 625-635.

McNicholas, W. T. (2000). Impact of sleep in COPD. *Chest, 117*, 48S-53S.

Mohsenin, V. (2007). Sleep in chronic obstructive pulmonary disease. *Sleep Medicine Clinics,* *2,* 1–8.

Rybarczyk, B., Stepanski, E., Fogg, L., Lopez, M., Barry, P., & Davis, A. (2005). A placebo-controlled test of cognitive-behavioral therapy for comorbid insomnia in older adults. *Journal of Consulting and Clinical Psychology, 73,* 1164–1174.

Kidney Disease

Chen, H. Y., Cheng, I. C., Pan, Y. J., Chiu, Y. L., Hsu, S. P., Pai, M. F., Yang, J.-Y., Peng, Y.-S., Tsai, T.-J., & Wu, K. D. (2011). Cognitive-behavioral therapy for sleep disturbance decreases inflammatory cytokines and oxidative stress in hemodialysis patients. *Kidney International, 80,* 415–422.

Chen, H. Y., Chiang, C. K., Wang, H. H., Hung, K. Y., Lee, Y. J., Peng, Y. S., Wu, K.-D., & Tsai, T. J. (2008). Cognitive-behavioral therapy for sleep disturbance in patients undergoing peritoneal dialysis: A pilot randomized controlled trial. *American Journal of Kidney Diseases, 52,* 314–323.

Hanley, P. (2008). Sleep disorders and end-stage renal disease. *Current Opinion in Pulmonary Medicine, 14,* 543–550.

Sabbatini, M., Pisani, A., Crispo, A., Ragosta, A., Gallo, R., Pota, A., Serio, V., Tripepi, G., & Cianciaruso, B. (2008). Sleep quality in patients with chronic renal failure: A 3-year longitudinal study. *Sleep Medicine, 9,* 240–246.

Alzheimer's Disease

Carter, P. A. (2006). A brief behavioral sleep intervention for family caregivers of persons with cancer. *Cancer Nursing, 29,* 95–103.

McCurry, S. M., Logsdon, R. G., Teri, L., & Vitiello, M. V. (2007). Sleep disturbances in caregivers of persons with dementia: Contributing factors and treatment implications. *Sleep Medicine Reviews, 11,* 143–153.

McCurry, S. M., Logsdon, R. G., Vitiello, M. V., & Teri, L. (2004). Treatment of sleep and nighttime disturbances in Alzheimer's disease: A behavior management approach. *Sleep Medicine, 5,* 373–377.

McCurry, S. M., Pike, K. C., Vitiello, M. V., Logsdon, R. G., Larson, E. B., & Teri, L. (2011). Increased walking and bright light exposure to improve sleep in community-dwelling persons with Alzheimer's disease: Results of a randomized, controlled trial. *Journal of the American Geriatrics Society, 59,* 1393–1402.

Vitiello, M. V., & Borson, S. (2001). Sleep disturbances in patients with Alzheimer's disease: Epidemiology, pathophysiology and treatment. *CNS Drugs, 15,* 777–796.

Parkinson's Disease

Claassen, D. O., & Kutscher, S. J. (2011). Sleep disturbances in Parkinson's disease patients and management options. *Nature and Science of Sleep, 3,* 125–133.

Comella, C. L. (2008). Sleep disorders in Parkinson's disease. *Sleep Medicine Clinics, 3,* 325–335.

Gagnon, J. F., Bédard, M. A., Fantini, M. L., Petit, D., Panisset, M., Rompré, S., Carrier, J., & Montplaisir, J. (2002). REM sleep behavior disorder and REM sleep without atonia in parkinson's disease. *Neurology, 59*, 585-589.

Iranzo, A., Molinuevo, J. L., Santamaria, J., Serradell, M., Marti, M. J., Valldeoriola, F., & Tolosa, E. (2006). Rapid-eye-movement sleep behaviour disorder as an early marker for a neurodegenerative disorder: A descriptive study. *Lancet Neurology, 5*, 572-577.

Schenck, C. H., Bundlie, S. R., & Mahowald, M. W. (1996). Delayed emergence of a parkinsonian disorder in 38% of 29 older men initially diagnosed with idiopathic rapid eye movement sleep behavior disorder. *Neurology, 46*, 388-393.

Tandberg, E., Larsen, J. P., & Karlsen, K. (1998). A community-based study of sleep disorders in patients with Parkinson's disease. *Movement Disorders, 13*, 895-899.

Multiple Sclerosis

Bamer, A. M., Johnson, K. L., Amtmann, D., & Kraft, G. H. (2008). Prevalence of sleep problems in individuals with multiple sclerosis. *Multiple Sclerosis, 14*, 1127-1130.

Stanton, B. R., Barnes, F., & Silber, E. (2006). Sleep and fatigue in multiple sclerosis. *Multiple Sclerosis, 12*, 481-486.

Veauthier, C., Radbruch, H., Gaede, G., Pfueller, C. F., Dörr, J., Bellmann-Strobl, J., Wernecke, K.-D., Zipp, F., Paul, F., & Sieb, J. P. (2011). Fatigue in multiple sclerosis is closely related to sleep disorders: A polysomnographic cross-sectional study. *Multiple Sclerosis Journal, 17*, 613-622.

CHAPTER 21

Baglioni, C., Battagliese, G., Feige, B., Spiegelhalder, K., Nissen, C., Voderholzer, U., Lombardo, C., & Riemann, D. (2011). Insomnia as a predictor of depression: A meta-analytic evaluation of longitudinal epidemiological studies. *Journal of Affective Disorders, 135*, 10-19.

Edinger, J. D., Olsen, M. K., Stechuchak, K. M., Means, M. K., Lineberger, M. D., Kirby, A., & Carney, C. E. (2009). Cognitive behavioral therapy for patients with primary insomnia or insomnia associated predominantly with mixed psychiatric disorders: A randomized clinical trial. *Sleep, 32*, 499-510.

Eidelman, P., Gershon, A., McGlinchey, E., & Harvey, A. G. (2012). Sleep and psychopathology. In C. M. Morin & C. A. Espie (Eds.), *The Oxford handbook of sleep and sleep disorders* (pp. 172-189). New York, NY: Oxford University Press.

Manber, R., Edinger, J. D., Gress, J. L., San Pedro-Salcedo, M. G., Kuo, T. F., & Kalista, T. (2008). Cognitive behavioral therapy for insomnia enhances depression outcome in patients with comorbid major depressive disorder and insomnia. *Sleep, 31*, 489-495.

Manber, R., Haynes, T., & Siebern, A. T. (2012). Sleep and psychiatric disorders. In C. M. Morin, & C. A. Espie (Eds.), *The Oxford handbook of sleep and sleep disorders* (pp. 471-501). New York, NY: Oxford University Press.

Morin, C. M., Stone, J., McDonald, K., & Jones, S. (1994). Psychological management of insomnia: A clinical replication series with 100 patients. *Behavior Therapy, 25*, 291-309.

Nappi, C. M., Drummond, S. P. A., & Hall, J. M. H. (2012). Treating nightmares and insomnia in posttraumatic stress disorder: A review of current evidence. *Neuropharmacology, 62,* 576-585.

Perlis, M. L., Sharpe, M., Smith, M. T., Greenblatt, D., & Giles, D. (2001). Behavioral treatment of insomnia: Treatment outcome and the relevance of medical and psychiatric morbidity. *Journal of Behavioral Medicine, 24,* 281-296.

Smith, M. T., Huang, M. I., & Manber, R. (2005). Cognitive behavior therapy for chronic insomnia occurring within the context of medical and psychiatric disorders. *Clinical Psychology Review, 25,* 559-592.

CHAPTER 22

Brzezinski, A., Vangel, M. G., Wurtman, R. J., Norrie, G., Zhdanova, I., Ben-Sushan, A., & Ford, I. (2005). Effects of exogenous melatonin on sleep: A meta-analysis. *Sleep Medicine Reviews, 9,* 41-50.

Hajak, G., Cluydts, R., Allain, H., Estivill, E., Parrino, L., Terzano, M. G., & Walsh, J. K. (2003). The challenge of chronic insomnia: Is non-nightly hypnotic treatment a feasible alternative? *European Psychiatry, 18,* 201-208.

Mayer, G., Wang-Weigand, S., Roth-Schechter, B., Lehmann, R., Staner, C., & Partinen, M. (2009). Efficacy and safety of 6-month nightly ramelteon administration in adults with chronic primary insomnia. *Sleep, 32,* 351-360.

Mendelson, W. B., Roth, T., Cassella, J., Roehrs, T., Walsh, J. K., Woods, J. H., Buysse, D. J., & Meyer, R. E. (2004). The treatment of chronic insomnia: Drug indications, chronic use and abuse liability. *Sleep Medicine Reviews, 8,* 7-17.

Meoli, A. L., Rosen, C., Kristo, D., Kohrman, M., Gooneratne, N., Aguillard, R. N., Fayle, R., Troell, R., Townsend, D., Claman, D., Hoban, T., Mahowald, M., Clinical Practice Review Committee, & American Academy of Sleep Medicine. (2005). Oral nonprescription treatment for insomnia: An evaluation of products with limited evidence. *Journal of Clinical Sleep Medicine, 1,* 173-187.

Morin, C. M., & Benca, R. (2012). Chronic insomnia. *The Lancet, 379,* 1129-1141.

National Institutes of Health. (2005). State of the Science Conference Statement on manifestations and management of chronic insomnia in adults, June 13-15, 2005. *Sleep, 28,* 1049-1057.

Roth, T., & Roehrs, T. (2010). Pharmacotherapy for insomnia. *Sleep Medicine Clinics, 5,* 529-539.

Sarris, J., & Byrne, G. J. (2011). A systematic review of insomnia and complementary medicine. *Sleep Medicine Reviews, 15,* 99-106.

Schneider-Helmert, D., & Spinweber, C. L. (1986). Evaluation of L-tryptophan for treatment of insomnia: A review. *Psychopharmacology, 89,* 1-7.

Schutte-Rodin, S., Broch, L., Buysse, D., Dorsey, C., & Sateia, M. (2008). Clinical guideline for the evaluation and management of chronic insomnia in adults. *Journal of Clinical Sleep Medicine, 4,* 487-504.

Sproule, B. A., Busto, U. E., Buckle, C., Herrmann, N., & Bowles, S. (1999). The use of nonprescription sleep products in the elderly. *International Journal of Geriatric Psychiatry, 14,* 851-857.

Taibi, D. M., Landis, C. A., Petry, H., & Vitiello, M. V. (2007). A systematic review of valerian as a sleep aid: Safe but not effective. *Sleep Medicine Reviews, 11*, 209–230.

Wade, A. G., Ford, I., Crawford, G., McConnachie, A., Nir, T., Laudon, M., & Zisapel, N. (2010). Nightly treatment of primary insomnia with prolonged release melatonin for 6 months: A randomized placebo controlled trial on age and endogenous melatonin as predictors of efficacy and safety. *BMC Medicine, 8*, 51.

Wilson, S. J., Nutt, D. J., Alford, C., Argyropoulos, S. V., Baldwin, D. S., Bateson, A. N., Britton, T. C., Crowe, C., Dijk, D.-J., Espie, C. A., Gringras, P., Hajak, G., Idzikowski, C., Krystal, A. D., Nash, J. R., Selsick, H., Sharpley, A. L., & Wade, A. G. (2010). British Association for Psychopharmacology consensus statement on evidence-based treatment of insomnia, parasomnias and circadian rhythm disorders. *Journal of Psychopharmacology, 24*, 1577–1601.

APPENDIX A

Ohayon, M. M., Carskadon, M. A., Guilleminault, C., & Vitiello, M. V. (2004). Meta-analysis of quantitative sleep parameters from childhood to old age in healthy individuals: Developing normative sleep values across the human lifespan. *Sleep, 27*, 1255–1273.

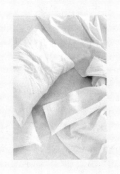

Appendix A

Sleep Stages and Cycles: The Basics

Your sleep diary provides good information about your sleep timing, quality, and quantity, and is the best way to measure sleep if you have insomnia. For more in-depth examination of sleep by scientists, or sleep medicine clinicians, special equipment is used to track sleep stages and cycles through the night. To determine sleep stages, three main measurements are used: brain waves, eye movements, and muscle tone. These are measured using electrodes that are attached to the scalp, the face near the eyes, and under the chin, respectively. The activity that is picked up by the electrodes is amplified and appears as wave forms on a screen. In the old days, the output from all the channels was printed by pens on big, folding chart paper that was moving at 30 mm per second through a polygraph. So, by morning, we had used lots of ink and almost half a mile's worth of chart paper! This huge stack of paper was then scored by flipping though the record and identifying the stages, page by page. Nowadays, the same information is collected and digitized by computer, and technologists score the record by viewing it on the computer screen rather than on paper.

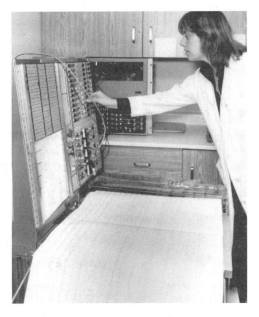

The author with a polygraph and moving chart paper to record sleep in the mid-1980s.

SLEEP STAGES

Wake

When we are awake, our brain waves are small and fast, mainly "beta" waves, which have a frequency of 12 cycles per second or more. As we become relaxed, we have more and more "alpha" waves, which are slower, at 8-12 cycles per second. While we are awake, our eyes are moving around a lot, and our muscle tension is high.

Stage 1 (N1)

As we become drowsy and are drifting off to sleep we enter Stage 1 (or N1 for non-REM sleep Stage 1), which is really a transitional stage between wake and sleep. We are in Stage 1 for a short time (1-7 minutes) before falling asleep. During Stage 1, in addition to alpha waves, our brain waves are slowing somewhat and we start having some "theta" waves, which have a frequency of 4-7 cycles per second. Our eyes don't dart around now; they start to roll slowly. Our muscle tone is still high.

Stage 2 (N2)

Stage 2 occurs when some specific wave forms called "spindles" and "K-complexes" appear. Spindles are spindle-shape clusters of waves that are 12-14 cycles per second. A K-complex is a large amplitude wave that occurs every so often. Between the spindles and the K-complexes are waves that are low amplitude and fast. Our eyes don't move very much in Stage 2 and muscle tone is lower than during Stage 1. When we reach Stage 2 sleep, we are considered to be officially asleep. We continue there for 10-25 minutes.

Stages 3 and 4 (Slow Wave Sleep, or N3)

As Stage 2 progresses, high amplitude slow waves occur more and more frequently. These are "delta" waves, which are slower than 4 cycles per second. When delta waves make up 20%-50% of the brain wave activity, Stage 3 is identified. Our eyes are not moving much and muscle tone is low. Stage 3 lasts just a few minutes and leads into Stage 4. Together, Stage 3 and Stage 4 are referred to as "deep" sleep, "delta sleep," or "slow wave sleep (SWS)." Stage 4 is just like Stage 3 except that it has a greater density of delta waves. When delta waves make up more than 50% of the activity, Stage 4 is identified. We are in Stage 4 for about 20-40 minutes at this point.

Rapid Eye Movement (REM) Sleep

After Stages 3 and 4, there is a brief "ascent" to Stage 2 before we enter the first REM period. REM is a distinct state, entirely different from the other ("non-REM") sleep stages.

Our brain waves are similar to those of wakefulness, with fast (beta wave) activity. Nearly all of our dreaming occurs in REM sleep. Our eyes dart around during bursts of activity (hence the name "rapid eye movement" sleep). These movements correspond to things we are seeing in our dreams. Unlike any other stage, our muscle tone is minimal. This is because all our postural muscles (the ones that allow movement to occur) are in a state of paralysis. Without this paralysis we would be acting out our dreams. The first REM period starts about 70-100 minutes after falling asleep, and it is short—about 1-5 minutes long.

Arousals

It is normal to move around and perhaps even wake up briefly before or after a REM period.

SLEEP CYCLES

The sequence of sleep stages I have just described represents the first sleep "cycle." We usually have about three more sleep cycles through the night, for a total of four. Each one is roughly 90–110 minutes long. The sleep stages occur in more or less the same order for each cycle. However, as the night goes on, we get less and less SWS per cycle and more and more REM sleep. By the end of the night we are spending most of our time in Stages 2 and REM.

SLEEP STAGE COMPOSITION OF A NIGHT'S SLEEP

The chart below gives you an idea of the relative amount of time spent in each stage of sleep over the whole night. It shows the total sleep duration and the percent of the night's sleep in each stage. Because these numbers change as we age, I am showing you representative data for a typical 20-year-old and a typical 60-year-old. You will see that there are three main differences between these two columns: The older person has a shorter sleep duration, more wakefulness during the night, and less SWS (deep sleep), than the younger person. Regardless of age, about half the night is spent in Stage 2 sleep and about one-fifth is in REM sleep.

	Age 20	Age 60
Total sleep time	7.5 hours	6.3 hours
Wake during the night	3%	10%
Stage 1	5%	6%
Stage 2	50%	54%
SWS (Stages 3 and 4)	20%	10%
REM	22%	20%

COMMON SLEEP MEASUREMENT TECHNIQUES

Sleep Diaries, as you've seen, are the measurement tool of choice for insomnia.

Polysomnography is measurement of sleep in the sleep lab, with electrodes that are attached to the scalp, face, and chin, to determine sleep stages. It also involves extra apparatus to check breathing, heart rhythm, blood oxygen levels, and limb movements. Polysomnography is the standard method of diagnosing sleep disordered breathing like sleep apnea, and some other sleep disorders like REM sleep behavior disorder and narcolepsy. It is *not* normally used for the evaluation of insomnia, unless there is a suspicion of another sleep disorder that can be picked up by polysomnography.

Actigraphy is another way that sleep can be measured, but only roughly. It is a movement sensor worn around the wrist like a watch. It collects data on movement over time. When there is a lot of movement, it is likely the person is awake; when there is little movement, it is likely the person is asleep. One of its benefits is that it can easily be used at home so a sleep lab stay is not required. However, it does not allow sleep stages to be identified so it is rarely used to diagnose sleep disorders. It can be useful for some types of sleep–wake research where there is no need for accurate measurement of sleep stages.

Portable monitors for so-called "home sleep tests" can be used to monitor airflow and breathing, but they don't usually monitor sleep stages. They are sometimes used to expedite the assessment of sleep disordered breathing when the sleep specialist strongly suspects that the person has obstructive sleep apnea.

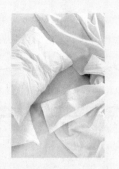

Appendix B
Extra Forms

Sleep Diary for the Week of: _____

DAY of the WEEK *Which night is being reported on?*		
Sleep timing		
1. I went to bed at *(clock time):*		
2. I turned out the lights after *(minutes):*		
3. I fell asleep in *(minutes):*		
4. I woke up ___ time(s) during the night. *(number of awakenings):*		
5. The total duration of these awakenings was *(minutes):*		
6. After awakening for the last time, I was in bed for *(minutes):*		
7. I got up at *(clock time):*		
Sleep quality — **The quality of my sleep was:** *1 = very poor; 10 = excellent*		
Naps *Number, time and duration*		
Alcohol *Time, amount, type*		
Sleep Medication *Time, amount, type*		
Notes:		

Bedtime: _____ **Rise Time:** _____

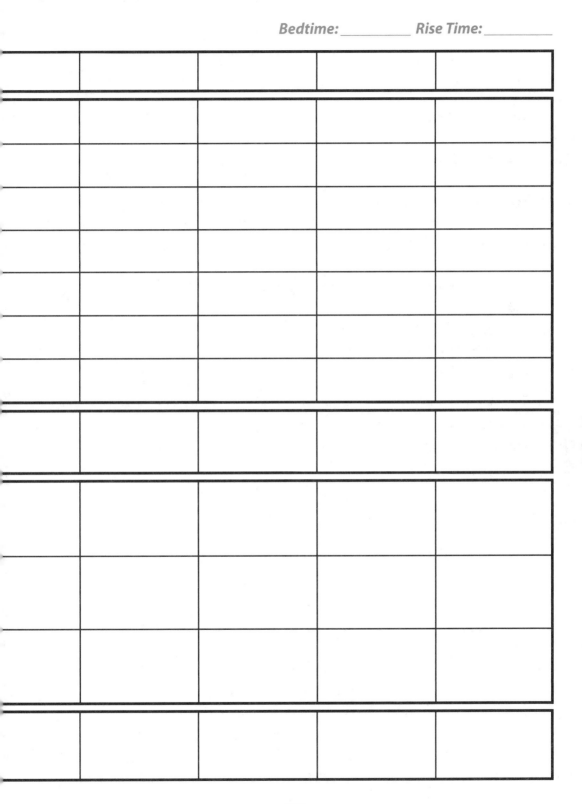

Sleep Diary for the Week of: _____

DAY of the WEEK *Which night is being reported on?*		

Sleep timing

1. **I went to bed at** *(clock time):*		
2. **I turned out the lights after** *(minutes):*		
3. **I fell asleep in** *(minutes):*		
4. **I woke up ___ time(s) during the night.** *(number of awakenings):*		
5. **The total duration of these awakenings was** *(minutes):*		
6. **After awakening for the last time,** **I was in bed for** *(minutes):*		
7. **I got up at** *(clock time):*		

Sleep quality

The quality of my sleep was: *1 = very poor; 10 = excellent*		

Naps *Number, time and duration*		
Alcohol *TIme, amount, type*		
Sleep Medication *TIme, amount, type*		

Notes:		

Bedtime: _____ **Rise Time:** _____

Calculating your Sleep Efficiency

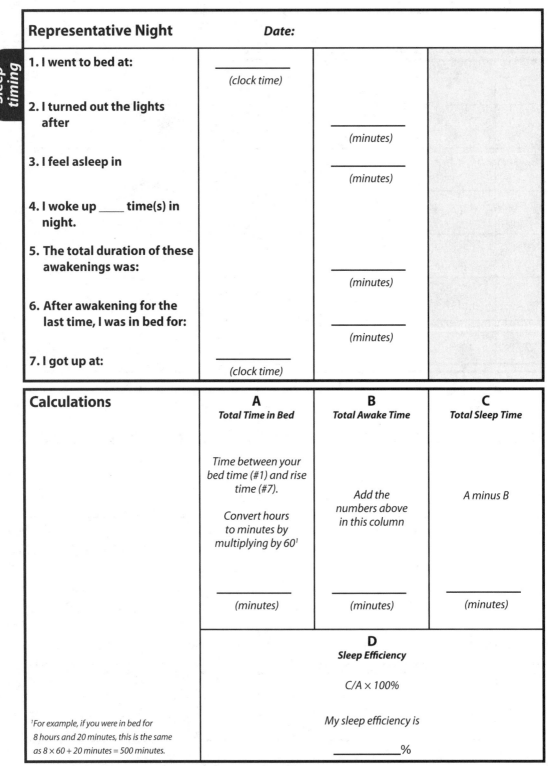

Representative Night	Date:		
1. I went to bed at:	_____ (clock time)		
2. I turned out the lights after		_____ (minutes)	
3. I feel asleep in		_____ (minutes)	
4. I woke up ____ time(s) in night.			
5. The total duration of these awakenings was:		_____ (minutes)	
6. After awakening for the last time, I was in bed for:		_____ (minutes)	
7. I got up at:	_____ (clock time)		

Calculations	**A** Total Time in Bed	**B** Total Awake Time	**C** Total Sleep Time
	Time between your bed time (#1) and rise time (#7). Convert hours to minutes by multiplying by 60[1]	Add the numbers above in this column	A minus B
	_____ (minutes)	_____ (minutes)	_____ (minutes)

D Sleep Efficiency
C/A × 100%
My sleep efficiency is
_____%

[1] For example, if you were in bed for 8 hours and 20 minutes, this is the same as 8 × 60 + 20 minutes = 500 minutes.

190

Calculating your Sleep Efficiency

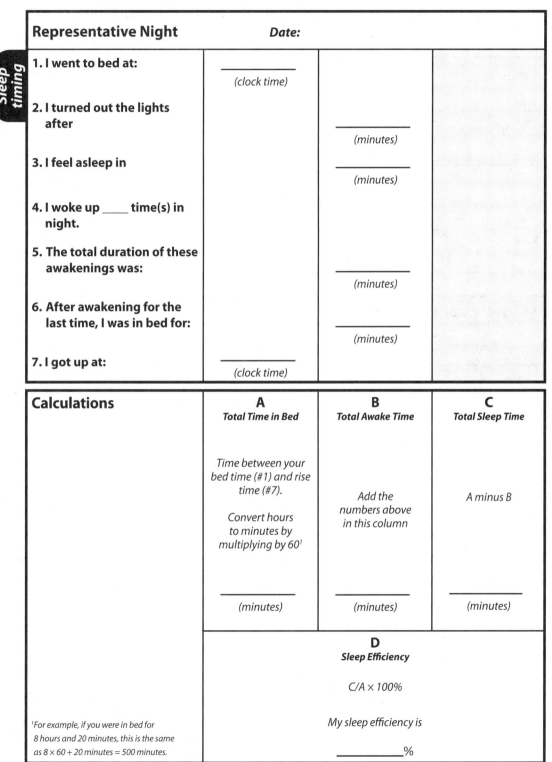

Sleep timing

Representative Night	Date:		
1. I went to bed at:	_____ *(clock time)*		
2. I turned out the lights after		_____ *(minutes)*	
3. I feel asleep in		_____ *(minutes)*	
4. I woke up ____ time(s) in night.			
5. The total duration of these awakenings was:		_____ *(minutes)*	
6. After awakening for the last time, I was in bed for:		_____ *(minutes)*	
7. I got up at:	_____ *(clock time)*		

Calculations	**A** *Total Time in Bed*	**B** *Total Awake Time*	**C** *Total Sleep Time*
	Time between your bed time (#1) and rise time (#7). *Convert hours to minutes by multiplying by 60[1]*	*Add the numbers above in this column*	*A minus B*
	_____ *(minutes)*	_____ *(minutes)*	_____ *(minutes)*

	D *Sleep Efficiency*
[1]*For example, if you were in bed for 8 hours and 20 minutes, this is the same as 8 × 60 + 20 minutes = 500 minutes.*	$C/A \times 100\%$ *My sleep efficiency is* _____%

Table for Adjusting Threshold Bedtime

Is your sleep efficiency...	If YES,
84% or less?	Set your threshold bedtime 15 minutes **later** this week.
85% to 89%?	Keep the **same** threshold bedtime this week.
90% to 94%?	Set your threshold bedtime 15 minutes **earlier** this week.
95% or greater?	Set your threshold bedtime 30 minutes **earlier** this week.

My **threshold bedtime** *and* **rise time**

    Bedtime: _____   **Rise time:** _____

Six Steps to Solid Sleep

1. Go to bed only when sleepy and not before your threshold bedtime. _____
   Fill in the threshold bedtime that you are setting for the upcoming week.

2. Maintain a regular threshold rise time in the morning. _____
   Fill in your threshold rise time (usually the same as before).

3. Use the bed only for sleeping. Sexual activity is the only exception. Do not watch television, listen to the radio, use electronic devices, eat, or read in bed.

4. Leave the bed if you can't fall asleep or go back to sleep within 10–15 minutes. Return when sleepy. Repeat this step as often as necessary during the night.

5. If sleepiness is overwhelming, you may take a short nap (no longer than 1 hour) in the afternoon, starting before 3 p.m.

6. Maintain a sleep diary.

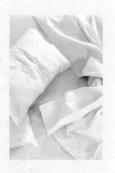

Index